# NeuroWisdom

### Bridging Neuroscience and Ancient Practices for Human Potential

**NeuroWisdom**

Bridging Neuroscience and Ancient Practices for Human
Potential

Copyright © *Levitas One*, 2024
All Rights Reserved

# What are the NoMAD Plans?

Developed by Dr Ash Kapoor, the NoMAD Plans represent a transformative approach to health and wellness that combines the wisdom of ancestral practices with contemporary medical insights. The name "NoMAD" not only suggests a journey through the intricate realm of health but also stands for its foundational principles: Nutritional Optimisation, Mindful Adaptation, and Detoxification.

At the heart of NoMAD is the 6 R Framework—Restore, Release, Repair, Renew, Reframe, and Represent. This methodology addresses the root causes of illness, combats chronic inflammation, and cultivates authentic vitality, guiding individuals through a transformative process.

Tailored specifically to each individual, NoMAD journeys are meticulously crafted to rebalance the body, strengthen the mind, and rejuvenate overall health. By integrating ancestral practices with cutting-edge, innovative treatments—all under strict medical oversight—NoMAD Plans offer a personalised pathway to sustainable, long-lasting well-being that resonates with your unique life circumstances.

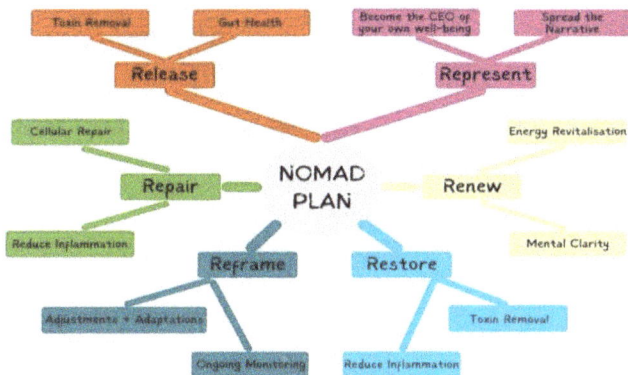

# Levitas One:
# "As Is In, As Is Out"

Reflecting the belief that our internal well-being is mirrored in our external environment. Founded by Dr. Ash Kapoor, Levitas One serves as the vehicle for delivering NoMAD's treatment plans. It envisions a healthcare future where patients are at the centre of a fully integrated, multidisciplinary approach. Guided by Nomads 6 Rs— Restore, Release, Repair, Renew, and Reframe, Represent— Levitas One empowers self-care through personalised guidance and minimal intervention, promoting long-term health, balance, and sustainability.

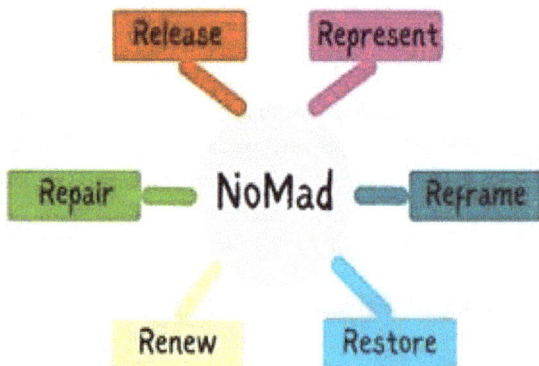

# Contents

# Preface

Over my nearly 35-year career as a physician, the last decade has transformed my understanding of human health and potential. My journey began in traditional medicine, but as I encountered more complex and chronic conditions, I realised that addressing symptoms alone was not enough. This led me down a path of root cause analysis—delving into the underlying dysfunctions that lie at the heart of illness.

What became increasingly clear is the undeniable power of the mind in shaping not only mental health but physical well-being. In patient after patient, I saw how unlocking the potential of the brain could change the trajectory of healing. From overcoming anxiety and chronic pain to enhancing cognitive performance and resilience, the brain became the central focus of my approach.

The insights in this book come from both scientific breakthroughs in neuroscience and the timeless wisdom of ancient practices. We stand at a unique intersection where technology and tradition converge, offering us tools to not only treat illness but optimise human potential. My experiences with patients have shown me that the brain is not just an organ to be studied but a powerful force that, when understood and nurtured, can transform lives.

This book is the culmination of my years exploring how neuroscience can be applied in everyday life to enhance health, resilience, and cognitive performance. It is my hope that the knowledge shared here will empower you to better understand your own brain, overcome limitations, and achieve your highest potential.

— *Dr Ash Kapoor*

# Introduction

## The Power of Neuroscience in Everyday Life

### Definition and Scope of Applied Neuroscience

Imagine your brain as a vast network of highways, each road representing a connection between neurons—cells that send and receive information. Now, what if we told you that these highways are constantly being built, expanded, and even rerouted? That's the power of **neuroplasticity**—the brain's ability to change and adapt in response to learning, experiences, and challenges. Applied neuroscience takes this understanding and translates it into practical tools for enhancing everyday life. Whether you are a student, an athlete, a professional, or simply seeking to improve your mental health, applied neuroscience can help you optimise your brain's function.

Neuroscience—the study of the brain and nervous system—was once limited to academic circles and complex laboratory research. However, recent advances have shown that the knowledge gained from neuroscience can be used to improve everyday experiences like learning new skills, managing stress, and even strengthening relationships. Applied neuroscience bridges the gap between theoretical science and real-world benefits by focusing on how the brain impacts behaviour, emotions, performance, and well-being.

Consider this: when we learn a new language, practice mindfulness, or recover from an injury, our brain physically changes. These changes happen at the level of neurons through processes called **synaptic plasticity** and **neurogenesis**, where new neural connections are formed and strengthened. Neuroscientists have mapped these processes, showing us how targeted exercises and behaviours can enhance cognitive flexibility, emotional regulation, and even physical health.

Applied neuroscience goes beyond the laboratory—it is about understanding these mechanisms and translating them into tools that anyone can use, whether to improve memory, combat depression, or develop leadership skills. Combined with insights from ancient wisdom, which offers time-tested approaches to health, balance, and personal growth, applied neuroscience becomes a powerful tool for everyone aged 18 to 70.

## *How Ancient Wisdom and Neuroscience Converge*

Though neuroscience is a relatively modern field, the brain's role in shaping our reality has been understood, albeit in different terms, for thousands of years. Ancient civilisations—whether through meditation, philosophical inquiry, or herbal medicine—have long recognised the connection between mind, body, and spirit. As modern neuroscience uncovers the mechanisms behind brain plasticity, emotional regulation, and cognitive function, it is becoming clear that much of what was practised in ancient cultures aligns with these scientific discoveries.

## 1. The Brain and Mindfulness: Ancient Practices Backed by Science

Take mindfulness, for example, a practice that originated over 2,500 years ago in Eastern traditions such as Buddhism. It emphasises present-moment awareness and calm focus. Neuroscientists now know that mindfulness meditation physically alters the brain. Studies show that regular meditation increases the thickness of the **prefrontal cortex**, the region responsible for decision-making and emotional control, and reduces the activity in the **amygdala**, the brain's fear centre. This helps people manage stress more effectively, just as ancient practitioners intended when they taught mindfulness for emotional balance.

A helpful analogy is to think of your brain as a muscle. Just as lifting weights strengthens your arms, practising mindfulness strengthens the connections in your brain that regulate attention and calm anxiety. Neuroscience explains the "how" behind the practice that ancient wisdom has long championed, creating a bridge between the two worlds.

## 2. The Gut-Brain Axis: Ancient Insights into Digestive Health

In ancient traditions like Ayurveda and Traditional Chinese Medicine, the link between digestion and mental clarity was widely understood. These systems viewed the gut as the seat of health and mental stability. Modern neuroscience confirms this through the study of the **gut-brain axis**—the bi-directional communication system between our gut and brain. A healthy gut microbiome supports the production of neurotransmitters like **serotonin**, which regulates mood. Disruptions in gut health can lead to mood disorders such as anxiety and depression.

By taking care of the gut through proper diet, herbs, and mindful eating practices—principles promoted by ancient wisdom—modern science now shows we can improve mental and emotional well-being. Just as ancient healers suggested that digestion impacts the mind, neuroscience shows us the direct pathways through which this occurs.

## 3. Neuroplasticity and Lifelong Learning: The Ancient Concept of a Flexible Mind

Ancient scholars like Aristotle believed in the concept of lifelong learning, promoting the idea that the mind can grow and change throughout life. Today, neuroplasticity—a core principle of modern neuroscience—proves that the brain can rewire itself at any age. Whether learning a new language, recovering from injury, or overcoming trauma, the brain can form new connections. This is why adults in their 60s or 70s can still learn to play an instrument or recover cognitive function after a stroke.

This convergence of ancient wisdom and neuroscience teaches us that flexibility is not just a mental exercise but a physical reality. When we engage in new learning or challenge ourselves, the brain grows—like a tree sprouting new branches. Ancient practices like yoga, meditation, and even creative arts were designed to cultivate this flexibility. Now, neuroscience confirms its profound effects on brain health and performance.

## 4. The Balance Between Left and Right Brain: Philosophical Insight Meets Science

In ancient philosophy, the balance between logic and creativity, or order and chaos, was seen as essential to well-being. This balance mirrors what modern neuroscience reveals about the **left and right hemispheres** of the brain. The left hemisphere is associated with logical thinking, language, and analysis. In contrast, the right hemisphere governs creativity, intuition, and visual-spatial skills. Too much dominance from one side can lead to an imbalance, making us overly analytical or too scattered. Practices like meditation or art, long prescribed by ancient traditions, help balance these two hemispheres, encouraging harmony between logic and creativity.

Neuroscience studies show that activities that engage both sides of the brain—such as learning a new skill, solving a puzzle, or practising mindfulness—help create stronger neural networks that boost cognitive performance and emotional resilience. Ancient wisdom, which encouraged activities promoting balance, was ahead of its time in understanding this crucial interplay.

### *Bridging Science, Clinical Practice, and Inspiration*

The beauty of applied neuroscience is that it does not just stay in the lab or the clinic—it is meant to inspire real-world transformation. Whether you are recovering from injury, struggling with mental health, or just wanting to optimise performance, applied neuroscience offers practical tools to improve your quality of life. When combined with the timeless wisdom of ancient practices, this approach becomes holistic, targeting not just the brain but the entire body and spirit.

Consider the case of someone recovering from a traumatic brain injury. Neuroplasticity allows the brain to repair itself, but recovery can be slow and frustrating. Adding mindfulness practices rooted in ancient traditions can accelerate this process by calming the nervous system, reducing stress hormones like **cortisol**, and promoting a healing environment in the brain. By integrating modern rehabilitation techniques with ancient mindfulness and holistic health approaches, we create a synergy that enhances recovery and overall well-being.

Similarly, in leadership or creativity, neuroscience teaches us how flow states—those moments of intense focus and productivity—are achieved. But ancient wisdom, whether through Zen meditation or Stoic philosophy, also offers insights into how to maintain a balanced and composed mind, essential for decision-making in high-pressure situations.

This book will guide you through these intersections of science and wisdom. Each chapter will offer actionable advice, scientific explanations, and real-world case studies to help you apply the lessons of neuroscience and ancient wisdom in your daily life. Whether you are striving for professional success, personal growth, or mental well-being, the power of the brain and the timeless knowledge of the past will provide the tools you need to thrive.

## Summary: Introduction

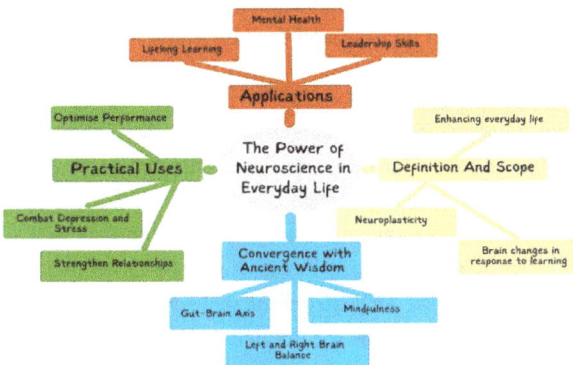

# Chapter 1
# The Structure of the Brain and Ancient Theories of Mind

## Neurons and Synaptic Connections

The human brain is a marvel of biological engineering, and neurons are its basic building blocks, much like bricks in a grand architectural structure or musicians in a well-tuned orchestra. Neurons communicate by sending electrical signals through synapses, which are tiny gaps between each neuron. This communication forms the intricate "wiring" of the brain, allowing us to think, feel, move, and interact with the world.

Imagine each neuron as a musician playing a unique note. Alone, that note does not amount to much. But when millions of neurons work together in harmony, they create a symphony of mental activity. Neurons work in concert through electrochemical signals, creating what we call neural networks. Synapses, the spaces between neurons, are like the gaps in an orchestra pit that the sound must bridge to reach the audience.

This connection gets stronger with practice. Think of it like exercising a muscle: the more you use specific neural pathways—whether it is learning a new skill, solving a puzzle, or practising mindfulness—the stronger the connection becomes. This process is known as *synaptic plasticity*. Just like how repetition makes a musician more adept at playing an instrument, repeatedly activating specific neural pathways strengthens the connections between neurons. Over time, these connections become more efficient, leading to enhanced learning and memory.

At the core of neuron communication are neurotransmitters, the chemicals that ferry signals between neurons. For instance, dopamine is involved in motivation and reward, while serotonin helps regulate mood. These neurotransmitters are like the different instruments in the orchestra, each adding a unique note to the overall symphony of brain function.

The science of neurons and synaptic connections has demystified much of the brain's complex activity. Understanding how these systems work allows us to appreciate the plasticity of our brains and to actively engage in practices that strengthen our cognitive abilities.

## Brain Regions and Functions

The brain is like a well-organised city, with various regions functioning as specialised departments. Each region of the brain has a role, from decision-making and problem-solving to emotional regulation and memory.

The *prefrontal cortex* can be thought of as the CEO of this bustling brain-city. Located at the front of the brain, it is responsible for decision-making, planning, and reasoning. This part of the brain is essential for tasks that require thought, like considering the consequences of an action, controlling impulses, or sticking to long-term goals. Whether it is deciding to save money rather than splurge or focusing on a work task without distraction, the prefrontal cortex is at work.

Next, we have the *hippocampus*, the brain's memory centre, which operates much like a librarian. It catalogues and organises information, helping us retain memories and recall facts. Whether you are remembering where you parked your car or studying for an exam, the hippocampus is working behind the scenes to ensure that information is stored and retrievable when needed.

The *amygdala*, meanwhile, serves as the brain's emotional hub. Located deep within the brain, the amygdala processes emotions such as fear, stress, and excitement. It acts like an alarm system, triggering a fight-or-flight response when faced with danger. However, when overstimulated—such as in chronic stress or anxiety—the amygdala can cause overreactions to everyday situations.

Interestingly, ancient civilisations also identified regions of the mind that had specialised functions. Traditional Chinese Medicine (TCM) believed the heart housed the "Shen" or spirit, responsible for consciousness and emotions. Ancient Greeks, like Plato and Aristotle, conceptualised the mind as having rational, emotional, and spirited parts—views that align remarkably with our modern understanding of the brain's regions and functions.

## Ancient Theories of Mind

Before the advent of neuroscience, ancient civilisations developed their own explanations for how the mind worked. Though their theories may seem primitive from a modern perspective, many of these ancient ideas closely mirror our current understanding of brain function.

In Ancient Egypt, for example, the heart was believed to be the centre of thought, emotion, and memory. The Egyptians saw the brain as relatively unimportant; in fact, they often discarded the brain during the mummification process, preserving the heart as the true seat of the soul. Though we now know that the brain controls cognition and emotion, the Egyptians' focus on the heart as a symbol of emotional balance and moral judgment echoes modern findings on the link between emotional health and physiological well-being.

In Ancient India, texts such as the *Upanishads* and the *Bhagavad Gita* conceptualised the mind as a battleground for different forces—desire, anger, wisdom, and peace. Achieving balance among these forces was seen as crucial to mental well-being, a notion not too distant from today's understanding of emotional regulation. Neuroscience now shows that balance in brain regions—such as the interaction between the emotional amygdala and rational prefrontal cortex—is essential for emotional and mental stability.

Plato and Aristotle also had theories about the mind. Plato divided the mind into three parts: the rational (located in the head), the spirited (in the chest), and the appetitive (in the stomach). According to Plato, the rational mind should govern the other parts to maintain harmony. This aligns with the modern understanding that the prefrontal cortex must regulate impulses and emotions originating from more primitive parts of the brain, such as the amygdala.

Although these ancient theories lacked scientific evidence, they recognised the mind's complexity in ways that resonate with today's neuroscience. By combining ancient insights with modern brain science, we can build a more holistic understanding of human consciousness and behaviour.

## Case Study and Practical Application

Consider the case of Sarah, a 45-year-old woman who suffered a stroke that left her unable to use her right arm and severely affected her memory. At first, Sarah felt like her life was over. Simple tasks had become difficult, and she felt overwhelmed by the prospect of recovery. However, through a combination of modern neuroscience techniques and ancient mindfulness practices, Sarah was able to rebuild her neural pathways and regain most of her lost abilities.

Following her stroke, Sarah worked with a neurologist who conducted brain imaging to determine the damage. The scans showed that parts of her *motor cortex* (responsible for movement) and *hippocampus* (responsible for memory) were damaged. Using the principles of neuroplasticity, Sarah's doctors prescribed a regimen of brain-training exercises designed to stimulate new neural connections. Tasks such as practising hand movements, memory exercises, and learning new skills were used to rewire her brain.

At the same time, Sarah began practising mindfulness meditation, a tradition rooted in ancient Buddhist practices. She learned to focus on her breath, observe her thoughts without judgment, and reduce her overall stress levels. This ancient practice helped her regulate her emotions and, more importantly, reduce the overactivity in her amygdala. By calming her stress response, Sarah was able to focus more effectively on her rehabilitation.

After months of combining brain-training with meditation, Sarah's brain began to form new neural connections to compensate for the areas damaged by the stroke. Her motor skills improved, and her memory gradually returned. Sarah's recovery demonstrates how modern neuroscience, in tandem with ancient wisdom, can lead to profound healing and cognitive improvement.

**Practical Tips:**

- **Neuroplasticity Exercises**: Engage in daily activities that challenge your brain, like learning a new instrument or solving puzzles, to strengthen neural connections.
- **Mindfulness Meditation**: Spend 10 minutes each day practising mindfulness to reduce stress and improve cognitive function.
- **Visualisation**: Use Visualisation techniques to mentally rehearse tasks or goals, activating both hemispheres of the brain for better performance and focus.

# Summary: The Structure of the Brain and Ancient Theories of Mind

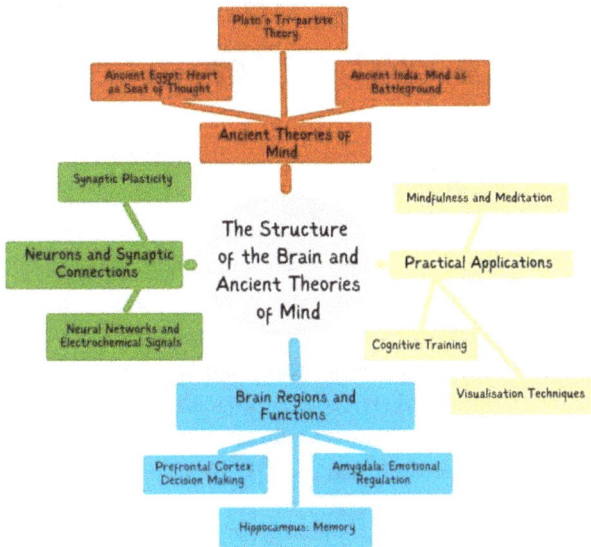

# Chapter 2
# Neuroplasticity, Cognitive Flexibility, and Ancient Learning Practices

## Scientific Research on Neuroplasticity

Neuroplasticity is the brain's remarkable ability to rewire itself in response to learning, experience, and even injury. Rather than being fixed and unchangeable, the brain is highly adaptable, constantly forming new neural pathways while pruning those that are underused. This adaptability is what allows us to learn new skills, recover from injuries like strokes, and even adapt to cognitive challenges. It is at the heart of cognitive flexibility—the brain's capacity to shift thinking, embrace new information, and solve problems creatively.

In earlier scientific understanding, it was believed that neurogenesis (the production of new neurons) ceased after early childhood. However, breakthroughs in research, particularly studies focusing on the hippocampus, have shown that neurogenesis continues well into adulthood. This discovery has far-reaching implications, proving that our brain remains malleable throughout life. In fact, activities such as learning new languages, playing musical instruments, or even engaging in brain-training exercises can enhance neural connections and foster new growth.

For instance, studies on stroke survivors have demonstrated that brain-training programs targeting affected areas can encourage the brain to form new connections. Patients who engage in specific exercises to stimulate motor or cognitive areas that were damaged have shown significant recovery in function. Similarly, adults learning a new language develop more robust neural pathways in regions related to memory and attention, underscoring that neuroplasticity enables us to continue growing cognitively well into old age.

The practical takeaway is that neuroplasticity empowers us to continuously improve our cognitive abilities. Whether it is learning a new skill, adopting a new habit, or recovering from injury, we can leverage the brain's inherent ability to adapt and rewire, turning everyday experiences into opportunities for cognitive enhancement.

## Ancient Learning Practices

Long before modern science discovered neuroplasticity, ancient cultures intuitively understood that the mind could be trained and shaped. These cultures developed methods that aligned closely with the principles of brain plasticity despite lacking the scientific language to explain their effectiveness.

In ancient Greece, intellectuals like Socrates and Aristotle emphasised the importance of mental training through debate, rhetoric, and philosophical inquiry. The Socratic method, which involved asking probing questions to challenge assumptions, fostered cognitive flexibility. This approach pushed students to engage in critical thinking, encouraging them to consider alternative perspectives and improve their reasoning abilities. Rhetorical debate not only demanded sharp memory and quick thinking but also exercised mental agility, a quality essential for both intellectual growth and practical problem-solving.

In India, the practices of yoga and meditation served as powerful tools for cultivating cognitive flexibility and emotional regulation. Yoga combined physical postures with focused breathing and concentration, providing a mental and physical discipline that heightened awareness and sharpened cognitive function. Meditation, on the other hand, was used to clear the mind and train focus. Ancient yogis believed that by mastering the mind, one could achieve mental clarity and wisdom. Today, modern neuroscience supports this ancient belief: studies show that meditation enhances grey matter density in the brain, particularly in regions associated with memory and emotional regulation.

Indigenous cultures worldwide used storytelling as a means of teaching and strengthening memory. Oral traditions, particularly those involving the recounting of long epics or histories, required tremendous mental discipline and engaged multiple parts of the brain. These cultures intuitively understood the power of narrative and memory, using stories to teach values, preserve history, and stimulate cognitive engagement. Modern neuroscience now recognises storytelling as a powerful tool that activates both hemispheres of the brain, improving both memory retention and cognitive flexibility.

These ancient practices demonstrate that humans have long understood the value of training the mind, even if they didn't have the scientific framework to explain why these practices worked. Today, we can see how these methods tapped into the brain's inherent plasticity, offering a wealth of wisdom to apply in our own pursuit of cognitive growth.

## Case Studies

The science of neuroplasticity has produced many remarkable stories of recovery and transformation, showing that the brain's capacity to change is far greater than previously believed. These case studies highlight how individuals have used neuroplasticity to overcome significant challenges and reshape their lives.

Consider David, a talented guitarist who suffered a traumatic brain injury after a car accident. His injury left him unable to use his right hand, seemingly ending his musical career. However, through intense rehabilitation and brain-training techniques, David was able to rebuild his neural pathways and regain his ability to play the guitar.

David's treatment involved mirror therapy—a method where the patient watches the reflection of their functioning limb in a mirror, tricking the brain into thinking the injured limb is moving. By combining mirror therapy with intense visualisation exercises, where

David imagined himself playing the guitar, he activated the same motor areas of his brain that had been damaged. Over time, these techniques helped David regain dexterity, and today, he is able to play music again. His case illustrates how focused brain training and neuroplasticity can help recover skills that seemed permanently lost.

Amy, a college student diagnosed with dyslexia, faced lifelong difficulties with reading and memory retention. However, by using neuroplasticity techniques, Amy was able to significantly improve her academic performance. She began by practising chunking—a strategy where information is broken down into smaller, manageable parts—and using mind maps, a visual tool to organise information. Over time, these methods helped rewire Amy's brain, enabling her to overcome her learning challenges. By engaging both hemispheres of her brain, she transformed her cognitive abilities, excelling in her studies and thriving in her academic environment.

These case studies demonstrate the power of neuroplasticity in helping individuals overcome seemingly insurmountable challenges. By understanding how the brain can adapt and rewire, anyone can harness its power to improve cognitive function, recover lost abilities, or enhance performance.

## Practical Tips

To harness the power of neuroplasticity and improve cognitive flexibility, here are some practical tips that blend modern neuroscience with ancient wisdom:

**Brain Training Games**: Engage in games and puzzles that challenge your brain, such as Sudoku, crossword puzzles, or chess. These activities stimulate neural growth and reinforce problem-solving pathways in the brain. Even modern apps like Lumosity or Peak can provide mental challenges to improve attention, memory, and cognitive flexibility.

**Learn Something New**: Whether it is picking up a new instrument, learning a language, or trying a new sport, challenging your brain with new activities helps strengthen neural connections. Each new skill requires different parts of the brain to work together, encouraging cognitive flexibility and promoting neurogenesis.

**Meditation for Mental Flexibility**: Daily mindfulness or meditation practices not only reduce stress but also improve focus and emotional regulation. Ancient wisdom holds that meditation sharpens the mind, and modern neuroscience confirms that it enhances the brain's ability to switch between tasks and adapt to new information.

**Physical Exercise**: Physical movement, especially aerobic exercise, boosts neurogenesis and improves overall brain health. Activities like walking, yoga, or swimming increase blood flow to the brain, helping to nourish neurons and support cognitive function. Regular exercise is also linked to improvements in memory and emotional regulation.

**Visualisation Techniques**: Use visualisation to enhance learning and performance. By mentally rehearsing a task, you activate the same neural pathways as if you were physically performing it. This technique is used by athletes, musicians, and even business professionals to boost performance.

By integrating these tips into daily life, you can actively engage your brain's plasticity and unlock your cognitive potential. Ancient practices like meditation and storytelling, combined with modern neuroscience techniques, provide a powerful toolkit for enhancing brain function at any age.

# Summary: Neuroplasticity, Cognitive Flexibility, and Ancient Learning Practices

# Chapter 3
# Depression, Mood, and Ancient Emotional Healing Practices

Depression is one of the most pervasive mental health challenges, affecting millions worldwide. It impacts mood, energy, motivation, and even physical health. While modern neuroscience has made significant strides in understanding depression, including its connection to brain chemistry, ancient civilisations developed their own methods of managing emotional distress. This chapter explores the science of neurotransmitters involved in mood regulation, examines ancient emotional healing practices, and presents case studies that demonstrate the intersection of ancient wisdom and modern mental health strategies. Finally, it offers practical tips for balancing mood using insights from both science and tradition.

## Neurotransmitters and Mood Regulation

Depression is often linked to imbalances in neurotransmitters, the brain's chemical messengers. The most prominent neurotransmitters associated with mood regulation are serotonin, dopamine, and norepinephrine. Understanding how these neurotransmitters function sheds light on the biological underpinnings of depression and the mechanisms behind treatments like antidepressants and lifestyle changes.

**Serotonin**: Often referred to as the "feel-good" neurotransmitter, serotonin plays a vital role in mood stabilisation, emotional well-being, and sleep regulation. Low levels of serotonin are strongly associated with depression, which is why many antidepressants (SSRIs) work by increasing serotonin levels in the brain. Serotonin also influences feelings of contentment and satisfaction, making it crucial for long-term emotional stability.

**Dopamine:** Dopamine is involved in the brain's reward system and is often linked to motivation, pleasure, and attention. In individuals with depression, dopamine levels are often reduced, leading to a lack of interest or pleasure in previously enjoyable activities (a condition known as anhedonia). Dopamine-boosting activities, such as exercise, creativity, or social interaction, are commonly recommended for improving mood and combating depression.

**Norepinephrine:** Known as the "fight-or-flight" chemical, norepinephrine helps regulate stress responses. In depression, norepinephrine levels can become dysregulated, leading to feelings of fatigue, apathy, and difficulty concentrating. Antidepressants like SNRIs (Serotonin-Norepinephrine Reuptake Inhibitors) aim to balance both serotonin and norepinephrine to alleviate these symptoms.

While these neurotransmitters play a central role in mood regulation, depression is not solely a chemical imbalance. It also involves emotional, cognitive, and social factors. Modern treatments combine pharmaceuticals with behavioural therapies, exercise, and diet to create a holistic approach. However, long before these scientific discoveries, ancient healing traditions recognised the importance of balance—between body, mind, and spirit—when treating emotional suffering.

## Ancient Wisdom in Emotional Healing

Ancient cultures had profound insights into emotional healing, and many of their practices, although lacking a modern scientific framework, aligned with principles we now understand about mood regulation and brain health.

**Ayurveda** (Ancient India): In Ayurvedic medicine, emotional balance is seen as a harmony between mind, body, and environment. Ayurveda emphasises the importance of managing stress and mental disturbances through lifestyle changes, diet, and meditation. Specific herbs like *Ashwagandha* and *Brahmi* were traditionally used to calm the nervous system and regulate mood. These herbs are now being studied for their adaptogenic properties, which help the body manage stress and anxiety by modulating the production of cortisol, an essential stress hormone.

**Traditional Chinese Medicine (TCM):** In TCM, emotions are believed to be intimately connected to specific organs—anger with the liver, grief with the lungs, and joy with the heart. Depression, often seen as a stagnation of energy (Qi), is treated by restoring balance through acupuncture, herbal remedies, and Qi Gong (a form of meditative movement). Acupuncture has been shown in modern studies to help release endorphins and regulate serotonin, providing scientific backing to these ancient practices.

**Buddhism** and **Mindfulness:** Long before mindfulness became a modern therapeutic practice, it was at the heart of Buddhist teachings. Meditation and mindfulness techniques were used to cultivate emotional awareness and detachment from negative thoughts. Research now supports the idea that mindfulness-based interventions (MBIs) improve mood and reduce symptoms of depression by increasing activity in the prefrontal cortex (the brain's executive function centre) and reducing activity in the amygdala (the fear and stress centre).

**Ancient Greek Philosophy:** The Stoics, such as Marcus Aurelius and Epictetus, emphasised emotional regulation through rational thought. They believed that suffering arises not from external events but from our perception of those events. This idea parallels modern cognitive-behavioural therapy (CBT), which teaches individuals to challenge and reframe negative thought patterns to improve emotional well-being.

**Shamanic Traditions:** Indigenous cultures worldwide used shamanic practices to treat emotional distress, often viewing depression as a soul imbalance. Rituals involving nature, music, and communal healing were central to restoring emotional equilibrium. Modern therapeutic approaches like music therapy and ecotherapy echo these ancient practices, highlighting the role of nature and rhythm in regulating mood.

These ancient methods remind us that emotional well-being is multifaceted, involving not just brain chemistry but also our connection to ourselves, our communities, and the natural world. Integrating these approaches with modern neuroscience offers a comprehensive pathway to healing.

## Case Studies

### Case Study 1: Sara's Recovery through a Holistic Approach

Sara, a 38-year-old woman, struggled with depression for most of her adult life. Despite trying several antidepressants, she found that her mood only improved slightly, and she often experienced side effects like fatigue and apathy. Frustrated, Sara turned to a more holistic approach, integrating modern and ancient practices to manage her depression.

She started a course of cognitive-behavioural therapy (CBT), which helped her challenge negative thought patterns, a core component of Stoic philosophy. She also incorporated mindfulness meditation into her daily routine, inspired by Buddhist teachings, which helped her become more aware of her emotions without being overwhelmed by them. Sara's therapist recommended she try acupuncture to complement her treatment, and she began weekly sessions. The acupuncture treatments helped her manage stress and improve her sleep quality.

Over time, Sara noticed significant improvements in her mood and energy levels. While she continued taking a low dose of antidepressants, it was the combination of CBT, mindfulness, and acupuncture that helped her find long-term relief. Sara's case highlights the power of combining modern science with ancient practices for a more holistic treatment of depression.

### Case Study 2: Mark's Experience with Meditation and Herbal Remedies

Mark, a 45-year-old corporate executive, experienced chronic stress and depression due to the high-pressure nature of his job. He found it difficult to relax, and his sleep suffered as a result. Mark decided to explore meditation, inspired by the rising popularity of mindfulness in the workplace. He began practising mindfulness meditation for 20 minutes every morning.

After a few weeks, Mark noticed a decrease in his anxiety and a more stable mood. Encouraged by this progress, he also began consulting with an Ayurvedic practitioner, who recommended taking Ashwagandha—a traditional herb known for its adaptogenic properties. Ashwagandha helped Mark manage his cortisol levels, the stress hormone that was contributing to his emotional imbalance. Over time, Mark found that he was not only more resilient in handling work stress, but his mood also improved significantly.

These case studies demonstrate how a combination of modern neuroscience and ancient healing traditions can offer a comprehensive approach to managing depression and stress.

## Practical Application

To improve emotional well-being and manage symptoms of depression, consider integrating modern neuroscience with ancient emotional healing practices. Here are practical steps and exercises that can be applied to your daily life:

### Mindfulness Meditation

Mindfulness has been scientifically proven to reduce symptoms of depression by increasing awareness of thoughts and emotions without becoming attached to them. Start with just 5–10 minutes a day of mindfulness practice. Focus on your breathing and gently bring your attention back whenever your mind wanders. Over time, this will help regulate the prefrontal cortex and reduce the activity of the amygdala, promoting emotional balance.

**Herbal Support**

Certain herbs, rooted in ancient traditions, have been shown to support mood and stress management. Consider incorporating **Ashwagandha** or **Rhodiola** into your routine. Both are adaptogens, which help balance cortisol and support the body's stress response. Always consult a healthcare provider before starting herbal supplements.

**Cognitive Behavioural Exercises (CBT)**

Inspired by Stoic philosophy and modern neuroscience, CBT involves identifying and challenging negative thought patterns. Start by writing down your negative thoughts, then ask yourself if these thoughts are rational or exaggerated. Reframe these thoughts with more balanced, constructive ones. Over time, this practice can help reshape neural pathways, leading to healthier emotional responses.

**Physical Activity**

Exercise is one of the most effective natural antidepressants. Physical activity increases serotonin and dopamine levels, improving mood and reducing stress. Incorporate at least 30 minutes of moderate exercise into your daily routine. Activities like yoga, which combines physical movement with mindfulness, are especially beneficial for both mental and physical health.

**Acupuncture**

If you are open to exploring ancient healing practices, acupuncture can be a valuable addition to your emotional wellness routine. Regular acupuncture sessions can help regulate neurotransmitters, promote relaxation, and improve sleep quality, all of which contribute to mood stabilisation.

By combining these modern and ancient practices, you can create a personalised approach to managing mood and depression, supporting both mental and physical well-being.

## Summary: Depression, Mood, and Ancient Emotional Healing Practices

# Chapter 4
# Anxiety, Stress, and Ancient Resilience-Building Practices

Anxiety and stress are widespread challenges in today's fast-paced world. Modern neuroscience has shed light on how these conditions affect the brain and body, but long before the advent of scientific research, ancient civilisations developed powerful practices to manage and build resilience against stress. By exploring the neuroscience of stress and anxiety alongside time-tested ancient wisdom, we can create a comprehensive approach to managing these conditions and enhancing our resilience in the face of life's challenges.

## Neuroscience of Stress

At its core, stress is the body's natural response to perceived threats or challenges. The brain is hardwired to respond to danger through the **fight-or-flight** mechanism, which is controlled by the **amygdala**— the brain's emotional processing centre. When the brain detects a threat, the amygdala triggers the release of stress hormones like **cortisol** and **adrenaline**, preparing the body to either confront the danger or flee from it. While this response is crucial for survival, prolonged or chronic stress can lead to significant mental and physical health issues, such as anxiety, depression, heart disease, and weakened immune function.

The key players in the stress response are the **hypothalamic-pituitary-adrenal (HPA) axis** and the **autonomic nervous system**. The HPA axis manages the release of cortisol, which helps regulate many of the body's processes, including metabolism, immune response, and memory. However, when cortisol levels remain elevated due to chronic stress, it can lead to long-term damage, affecting brain regions such as the **hippocampus** (responsible for memory) and **prefrontal cortex** (involved in decision-making and impulse control).

This overexposure to cortisol can result in **impaired cognitive function**, emotional instability, and a higher risk of anxiety disorders.

Stress also activates the **sympathetic nervous system**, which increases heart rate, blood pressure, and muscle tension, all of which prepare the body for action. In contrast, the **parasympathetic nervous system** helps to calm the body down after a stressful event, returning it to a state of rest and recovery. However, people who experience chronic stress often have difficulty activating this calming system, leading to ongoing feelings of anxiety and tension.

**Anxiety**, which is often triggered by stress, involves heightened activity in the amygdala and reduced regulation from the prefrontal cortex. This imbalance causes individuals to experience overwhelming feelings of fear, worry, and hypervigilance, even in situations where there is no immediate threat. Anxiety can also interfere with the brain's ability to differentiate between real and perceived threats, further fueling the cycle of worry.

Neuroscience has shown that stress and anxiety affect not only the brain but also the **body's immune system** and **gastrointestinal function**, leading to a range of physical symptoms such as headaches, digestive issues, and fatigue. Fortunately, modern science has begun to validate ancient practices that can help regulate the brain's stress response and build resilience.

## Ancient Resilience Practices

Before the era of brain scans and psychological research, ancient cultures around the world had already developed profound practices to manage stress and build emotional resilience. These techniques were often intertwined with spiritual, physical, and communal life, offering a holistic approach to maintaining well-being. While they may have lacked scientific terminology, these practices align closely with what modern neuroscience now understands about regulating the nervous system and managing stress.

**Yoga and Pranayama (Ancient India):** The ancient practice of **yoga**, which originated in India over 5,000 years ago, was designed not only to improve physical health but also to calm the mind and balance the body's energy. One of the critical components of yoga is **pranayama** (breath control), which has been shown to reduce stress and anxiety by activating the **parasympathetic nervous system**. Breathwork practices, such as **alternate nostril breathing** and **deep diaphragmatic breathing**, help regulate the heart rate and reduce cortisol levels. Modern studies show that pranayama enhances oxygenation of the brain, improves emotional regulation, and lowers anxiety.

**Meditation and Mindfulness (Buddhism and Hinduism):** Meditation practices, central to both **Buddhist** and **Hindu** traditions, were designed to train the mind to achieve emotional balance, mental clarity, and inner peace. **Mindfulness meditation**, which involves focusing on the present moment without judgment, is particularly effective in managing stress. Neuroscience has confirmed that regular meditation reduces the activity of the **amygdala**, decreases cortisol production, and strengthens the **prefrontal cortex**, allowing for better emotional regulation and decision-making in stressful situations.

**Qi Gong and Tai Chi (Traditional Chinese Medicine):** In ancient China, **Qi Gong** and **Tai Chi** were developed as systems to harmonise the body, mind, and spirit. These slow, deliberate movements, combined with focused breathing, are designed to cultivate **Qi** (life energy) and promote balance. Modern research shows that these practices help reduce anxiety by improving heart rate variability (HRV), which reflects the balance between the sympathetic and parasympathetic nervous systems. By enhancing the body's ability to switch between stress response and relaxation, these ancient techniques build resilience to life's challenges.

**Stoicism (Ancient Greece):** The **Stoics** of ancient Greece, such as **Epictetus** and **Marcus Aurelius**, believed that emotional resilience comes from accepting what is within our control and letting go of what is not. This philosophy aligns with the principles of **cognitive-behavioural therapy (CBT)**, a modern psychological practice that helps people reframe negative thoughts and reduce anxiety. Stoicism teaches individuals to remain calm under pressure by focusing on rational thought, which helps regulate emotional responses—a concept that modern neuroscience confirms as effective for stress management.

# Case Studies

### Case Study 1: Laura's Journey from Anxiety to Calm

Laura, a 28-year-old graphic designer, had always struggled with anxiety, especially when meeting deadlines at work. Her constant worrying about her performance and fear of criticism often left her feeling overwhelmed and physically exhausted. After trying various therapies with limited success, Laura decided to incorporate ancient practices into her life to help manage her stress more effectively.

She began practising yoga, specifically **Vinyasa Flow**, three times a week, combining physical movement with mindful breathing exercises. Over time, Laura noticed a significant reduction in her anxiety levels, as the deep breathing activated her parasympathetic nervous system, helping her calm down after stressful days. Encouraged by this progress, she added **mindfulness meditation** to her morning routine, spending 10 minutes focusing on her breath and letting go of negative thoughts. This practice helped rewire her brain to reduce activity in her amygdala and strengthen her prefrontal cortex, improving her ability to manage stress without becoming overwhelmed.

Within a few months, Laura was not only meeting her deadlines with less anxiety but also enjoying her work more. By integrating ancient practices with modern mindfulness techniques, Laura built resilience to stress and improved her overall quality of life.

### Case Study 2: Robert's Use of Stoic Philosophy to Combat Work Stress

Robert, a 45-year-old entrepreneur, faced immense pressure running his own business. He often felt anxious about the future of his company and worried constantly about factors outside of his control, such as market fluctuations and client demands. This chronic stress started to affect his health, leading to insomnia and digestive issues.

Inspired by a friend, Robert began reading about **Stoicism**. He was particularly struck by the teachings of **Epictetus**, who emphasised the importance of focusing on what is within one's control and letting go of what isn't. Robert started incorporating Stoic practices into his daily routine, including **morning reflection**, where he mentally prepared for the challenges of the day by reminding himself to focus only on his actions, not external outcomes.

By adopting this mindset, Robert was able to reduce his stress levels significantly. He no longer felt overwhelmed by things he couldn't control and instead focused on making the best decisions in the moment. This shift in perspective helped him manage his stress more effectively and improved his emotional resilience. Over time, he also incorporated **deep breathing exercises** from **Tai Chi** to calm his nervous system, creating a balanced approach to managing work stress.

## Practical Application

Here are some practical, actionable steps that integrate neuroscience with ancient resilience practices to help manage anxiety and stress:

1. **Mindful Breathing**: Practice **deep diaphragmatic breathing** or **pranayama** techniques to activate your parasympathetic nervous system. Start by inhaling deeply through your nose for 4 seconds, holding for 4 seconds, and exhaling through your mouth for 6 seconds. Repeat this cycle 5–10 times whenever you feel stressed to lower cortisol levels and calm your nervous system.

2. **Daily Meditation**: Spend at least 10–15 minutes each day practising **mindfulness meditation**. Focus on your breath, gently bringing your attention back whenever your mind wanders. This practice helps reduce activity in the amygdala, the brain's fear centre and promotes better emotional regulation. Over time, this will build resilience to stress.

3. **Physical Movement**: Incorporate practices like **yoga, Qi Gong**, or **Tai Chi** into your weekly routine. These practices combine movement with breath, helping to balance the autonomic nervous system and reduce anxiety. Even 15–30 minutes a day can have a profound impact on your ability to manage stress.

4. **Cognitive Reframing**: Adopt a **Stoic mindset** by regularly reflecting on what is within your control and what is not. Practice letting go of external outcomes and focusing on your actions and decisions in the moment. This cognitive shift, similar to **CBT**, helps reduce the mental burden of worrying about things you cannot change.

5. **Journaling**: At the end of each day, reflect on moments of stress and how you responded. Use this time to practise gratitude and recognise how you successfully managed challenges. This simple act of reflection helps train the brain to focus on positive outcomes and build emotional resilience.

By combining modern neuroscience with the time-honoured wisdom of ancient practices, you can effectively manage anxiety and stress, building resilience that supports both mental and physical well-being over the long term.

# Summary: Anxiety, Stress, and Ancient Resilience-Building Practices

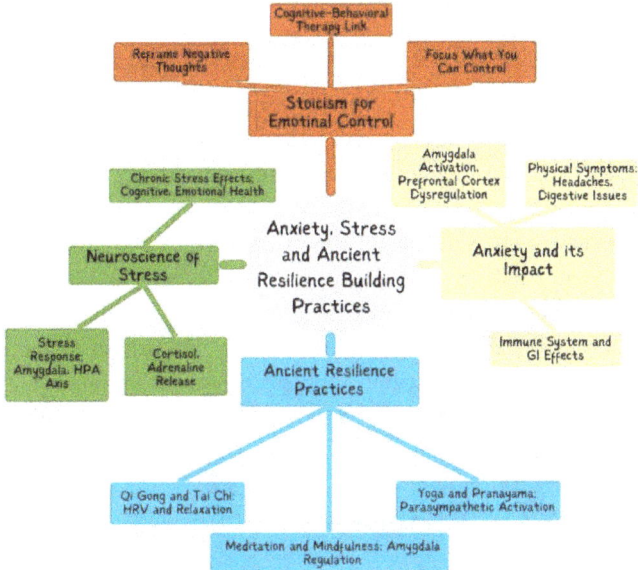

# Chapter 5
# How We Learn and Ancient Memory Systems

Learning and memory are central to human experience. Our ability to absorb information, recall details, and apply knowledge in new contexts shapes how we navigate life. Neuroscience has greatly advanced our understanding of how memory is formed and stored in the brain. Still, ancient cultures also developed sophisticated mnemonic systems to enhance memory long before modern science could explain the brain's processes. This chapter explores how learning and memory occur in the brain, examines ancient techniques used to strengthen memory, and provides practical tips for optimising memory in everyday life.

## Memory Formation and the Hippocampus

Memory is a complex process involving several brain regions, but the **hippocampus** plays a critical role in consolidating new information into long-term memories. This small, seahorse-shaped structure, located in the **temporal lobe**, acts like a librarian, organising and filing away new memories for future retrieval.

Memory formation begins with **encoding**, where sensory information (what you see, hear, or feel) is processed by the brain. This information is then stored temporarily in short-term memory. If deemed important enough, it is transferred to long-term memory through **consolidation**, a process primarily governed by the hippocampus. During consolidation, neural connections are strengthened, allowing the memory to become more stable and durable over time. Studies have shown that sleep is vital for this consolidation process, as the brain uses sleep to reorganise and strengthen synaptic connections.

The hippocampus is also deeply involved in **spatial memory**, which helps us navigate environments and remember locations. This is why ancient mnemonic techniques, which often rely on the visualisation of spatial environments (like the **Memory Palace**), are so effective at enhancing memory.

Memory retrieval, the final step in the process, depends on the strength and accessibility of the neural pathways formed during consolidation. The more frequently you recall a memory or engage with information, the stronger these pathways become, making it easier to retrieve that memory in the future. This phenomenon explains why repetition and active recall are critical strategies for improving long-term memory retention.

However, memory is not flawless. Over time, neural pathways may weaken if a memory isn't regularly revisited, leading to **forgetting**. Additionally, the brain's capacity for **neuroplasticity**—its ability to form new connections and reorganise itself—means that old memories can sometimes be altered or distorted as new information is learned.

Modern neuroscience emphasises the importance of **synaptic plasticity** in memory formation—the brain's ability to strengthen the connections between neurons in response to learning. Key neurotransmitters like **glutamate** and **acetylcholine** are involved in enhancing these connections, playing a major role in how well we remember information over time.

## Ancient Mnemonic Techniques

Long before the advent of scientific research into memory, ancient cultures developed powerful mnemonic techniques to enhance memory retention. These systems, though rooted in different cultural practices, often employed similar principles: visualisation, spatial memory, and the association of abstract information with vivid imagery.

**The Memory Palace (Method of Loci)**

One of the oldest and most effective memory techniques is the **Memory Palace,** also known as the **Method of Loci.** This technique originated in ancient Greece and was famously used by Greek and Roman orators to deliver long speeches without notes. The method involves a familiar place (like your home or a palace) and mentally placing items or concepts you want to remember in specific locations within this environment. By walking through the space in your mind, you can recall each item or piece of information by visualising where you "placed" it. This technique leverages the brain's natural strength in **spatial memory,** a vital function of the hippocampus, making it easier to retain and retrieve information.

**The Art of Memory (Medieval Europe)**

In medieval Europe, scholars and monks used a variation of the Memory Palace technique, often referred to as the **Art of Memory.** This system used cathedrals or religious imagery as memory aids. For example, monks would mentally place scriptures or prayers in specific locations within a cathedral or church. The vivid visual and emotional associations helped them retain large volumes of religious text, which was essential in an age when written texts were rare.

**Storytelling and Oral Tradition (Indigenous Cultures)**

In many indigenous cultures, storytelling was both an art form and a vital method for transmitting knowledge. Epic stories, myths, and genealogies were passed down through generations, often without any written records. These oral traditions employed repetition, rhythm, and emotional content to make the stories more memorable. In ancient India, for example, **Vedic scholars** memorised entire religious texts by heart using rhythmic chants and repetitive vocal patterns. These techniques engaged multiple areas of the brain, including auditory and emotional centres, making the material easier to recall.

### The Peg System (Ancient China)

Another ancient technique is the **Peg System**, which was used in ancient China and has since been adopted worldwide. This method involves associating numbers with specific, easily visualised objects or images (known as pegs). For example, if you need to remember a grocery list, you could associate the number one with a tree and imagine apples hanging from its branches. This method relies on the brain's ability to create strong associations between numbers and visual images, facilitating easier recall.

These ancient mnemonic systems not only enhanced memory but also aligned with what we now know about **neuroplasticity** and the brain's capacity for learning through repetition, Visualisation, and emotional engagement. By connecting abstract concepts to concrete, emotionally charged images, these techniques activate multiple brain regions, making information more memorable.

# Case Studies

### Case Study 1: The Modern Use of the Memory Palace

Consider the story of **Dominic O'Brien**, an eight-time World Memory Champion, who used the **Memory Palace** technique to Memorise the order of 54 shuffled decks of playing cards. O'Brien's method involved associating each card with a vivid, unusual image and then placing these images in specific locations within an imagined environment. By mentally walking through his Memory Palace, O'Brien was able to recall each card in order—a remarkable feat of memory that neuroscience explains through the activation of the hippocampus and visual processing areas of the brain.

Modern brain imaging studies have shown that memory champions like O'Brien do not necessarily have larger hippocampi or better innate memory than others. Instead, they use more efficient memory strategies—leveraging visual imagery and spatial memory, much like the ancient Greeks and Romans did with the Method of Loci.

## Case Study 2: Oral Tradition in Indigenous Cultures

In indigenous cultures, oral storytelling has played a crucial role in preserving history, culture, and knowledge. The **Māori** people of New Zealand, for example, have long used oral traditions to pass down genealogies, historical events, and cultural wisdom. These stories are often recited with great emotional intensity and vivid imagery, which helps embed them deeply in the memory of both the storyteller and the listeners. Neuroscience has shown that emotional engagement strengthens memory retention by activating the amygdala, which enhances the consolidation of memories in the hippocampus.

The transmission of these stories has been so effective that many Māori can trace their family lineage back several centuries. This tradition demonstrates how the brain can retain vast amounts of complex information when it is encoded using emotionally charged, structured narratives.

## Case Study 3: Dyslexia and the Peg System

**Sarah**, a high school student with dyslexia, struggled with memorising numbers and sequences, which made subjects like math particularly challenging. Her tutor introduced her to the **Peg System**, teaching her to associate each number with a vivid image (e.g., 1 = sun, 2 = shoe, 3 = tree). By using this system, Sarah was able to create mental images of the numbers she needed to remember. Over time, this technique helped her overcome her learning challenges by strengthening the neural connections involved in visual and spatial memory.

Neuroscience research supports the use of visual mnemonic systems for students with learning disabilities, as they can engage different parts of the brain to compensate for difficulties in traditional learning methods. Sarah's success in math was a direct result of using the brain's natural capacity for **neuroplasticity**, aided by ancient memory techniques.

# Practical Tips

To improve your own memory and learning abilities, you can integrate both modern neuroscience-backed strategies and ancient mnemonic techniques. Here are practical tips to get you started:

## Use the Memory Palace Technique

Choose a familiar place, such as your home, and imagine yourself walking through it. As you move from room to room, mentally place items or information you need to remember in each location. When it is time to recall the information, mentally walk through your Memory Palace to retrieve the details. This technique is highly effective for remembering lists, names, or even complex information-like speeches.

## Visualise to Memorise

When learning something new, try to create vivid mental images that represent the information. The more unusual or emotionally charged the image, the easier it will be to remember. For example, if you are trying to remember a historical date, imagine a scene from that era with exaggerated characters and details.

## Leverage Repetition and Active Recall

Studies show that repetition strengthens neural connections. To retain information, regularly review what you've learned using **spaced repetition**, where you revisit the material at increasing intervals. **Active recall**—the process of testing yourself without looking at the material—also helps reinforce memory by making the brain actively retrieve the information.

## Meditation and Focus:

Incorporate short sessions of mindfulness or meditation into your routine to enhance focus and cognitive clarity. Meditation has been shown to increase grey matter in regions associated with memory and emotional regulation, improving your brain's ability to consolidate and retain information.

## Mind Maps and Chunking

Break down complex information into smaller chunks or groups. This technique, known as **chunking**, makes the material easier to process. You can also use **mind maps** to visually organise information, linking concepts in a way that mimics the brain's natural associative networks.

By combining these practical tips with insights from both neuroscience and ancient wisdom, you can optimise your learning, strengthen your memory, and improve cognitive performance in both your personal and professional life.

## Summary:How We Learn and Ancient Memory Systems

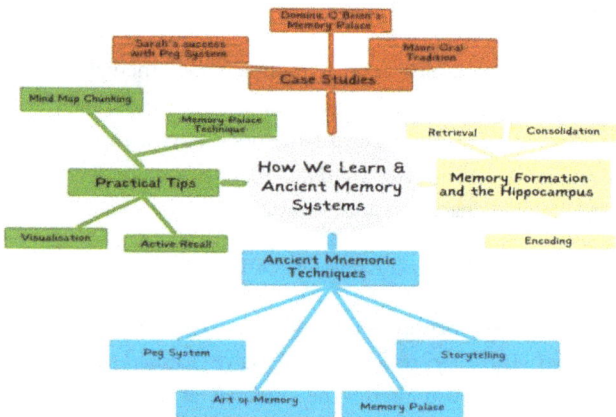

# Chapter 6
# Enhancing Cognitive Performance with Focus and Ancient Flow States

Focus and the ability to enter a state of flow are central to cognitive performance. Neuroscience has begun to unlock the mechanisms that allow us to concentrate deeply on tasks, while ancient cultures developed their own methods for cultivating flow—a state of effortless engagement where distractions disappear and performance peaks. This chapter explores the neuroscience behind the focus, delves into ancient techniques for achieving flow, and provides real-world case studies and practical tips for integrating these insights into everyday life.

## The Neuroscience of Focus

At the core of cognitive performance is our ability to focus—directing sustained attention toward a specific task while filtering out distractions. Neuroscientifically, focus is managed primarily by the **prefrontal cortex**, the brain's control centre for executive functions like decision-making, goal-setting, and sustained attention. When we focus, this region works with other parts of the brain, like the **parietal cortex** (responsible for spatial attention) and **thalamus** (which filters sensory information), to concentrate our mental energy on the task at hand.

**Neurotransmitters** play a crucial role in maintaining focus. **Dopamine**, a key neurotransmitter, is involved in motivation and reward, helping to keep us engaged in tasks we find challenging or enjoyable. **Norepinephrine**, another neurotransmitter, increases alertness and focus, heightening our attention to detail. When these chemicals are in balance, the brain can enter a state of heightened concentration, allowing for optimal performance.

However, the brain is naturally wired to seek out new stimuli—something we can trace back to evolution when our survival depended on quickly noticing changes in our environment. This creates a challenge in today's world, where digital distractions constantly compete for our attention. **Multitasking**, often seen as a desirable skill, is actually counterproductive in most cases, as the brain isn't wired to focus on more than one complex task at a time. Every time we switch between tasks, the brain must reset, leading to **cognitive fatigue** and reduced efficiency.

Focus is also limited by the **attentional span**, which varies among individuals. Research suggests that after about 90 minutes of intense focus, cognitive performance begins to decline, making breaks essential for maintaining long-term productivity.

**Neuroplasticity** allows us to train and improve our focus over time. Just as athletes train their muscles, we can train our brains to maintain longer periods of concentration. Mindfulness practices, which help strengthen the prefrontal cortex, have been shown to enhance sustained attention. In fact, studies reveal that as little as 10 minutes of mindfulness meditation a day can significantly improve focus and attention.

## Ancient Flow Techniques

Long before neuroscience could explain the mechanics of focus, ancient cultures developed methods to enter what we now call a **flow state**—a condition of total immersion in an activity. In flow, a person becomes so deeply absorbed that time seems to disappear, and performance reaches its peak. Flow states, while common in activities like sports, music, and art, are achievable in any field where skill meets challenge.

The concept of flow aligns with ancient techniques found in various cultures, where achieving a state of **effortless focus** was often associated with spiritual or philosophical practices.

**Zen Buddhism** developed the idea of **mushin** or "no-mind," where the mind is completely free from distractions and emotional clutter, allowing an individual to act effortlessly and intuitively. This state was cultivated by **samurai warriors** during swordsmanship training. The goal was to react without thinking, relying on muscle memory and heightened awareness. Modern neuroscience suggests that during flow, the **prefrontal cortex** temporarily quiets down, leading to reduced self-criticism and doubt, which allows performance to feel more automatic and smooth.

In ancient **Greek culture**, the concept of **arête** (excellence) was tied to achieving peak performance through the integration of body and mind. Greek athletes and scholars alike engaged in activities like running, wrestling, and philosophy with the goal of reaching their personal best. Flow was achieved by aligning one's skills with the challenge at hand—whether in a physical competition or intellectual debate.

In **Indian yoga** traditions, achieving **dhyana** (deep meditation) was a way to focus the mind and enter a state of flow. Through **asana** (physical postures) and **pranayama** (breath control), practitioners could calm the mind and body, setting the stage for deep concentration. Modern research confirms that yoga and controlled breathing help regulate the **autonomic nervous system**, promoting a state of calm and focus conducive to flow.

Ancient **indigenous cultures** also used storytelling, dance, and rhythmic drumming to enter flow states. These activities required participants to fully immerse themselves, allowing creativity and movement to emerge naturally. Neuroscientific research on rhythmic activities like drumming shows that these practices synchronise brain waves, particularly in the **alpha** and **theta** ranges, associated with deep relaxation and creative problem-solving.

All of these ancient flow techniques have parallels in modern flow science, which emphasises the importance of balancing challenge with skill, maintaining intrinsic motivation, and eliminating distractions to enter this optimal state of performance.

# Case Studies

### Case Study 1: Mihaly Csikszentmihalyi and Modern Flow Theory

Mihaly Csikszentmihalyi, a Hungarian-American psychologist, is one of the most influential modern thinkers on flow states. His research in the 1970s led to the discovery that people feel happiest and perform best when they are fully absorbed in what they are doing. Whether playing chess, climbing mountains, or painting, people entering a flow state experience a sense of timelessness and deep satisfaction.

One study Csikszentmihalyi conducted involved analyzing **chess players**. The players reported that when they were deeply engaged in the game, all distractions faded away, and they became fully immersed in the task. Brain scans show that during this kind of focus, the **prefrontal cortex**—which governs self-awareness and doubt— quieted down, allowing for smoother, more intuitive decision-making.

Csikszentmihalyi's work revolutionised how we understand high performance and mental well-being, showing that flow is accessible to anyone in almost any field when conditions are right: a clear goal, intrinsic motivation, and a balance between the challenge and one's skills.

### Case Study 2: Flow in Martial Arts

In ancient **Japanese martial arts**, the concept of **mushin** (no-mind) was essential for mastery. One famous samurai, **Miyamoto Musashi**, described this state in his writings. In battle, a samurai could not afford to be distracted by emotions, fear, or overthinking. Instead, they trained to act reflexively, relying on their skills without conscious thought. Musashi's approach involved continuous practice and mindfulness, allowing him to develop the ability to enter flow on demand.

Modern martial artists also report flow states during competition. Studies on **Brazilian Jiu-Jitsu practitioners** show that when athletes are in flow, their perception of time slows down, their movements become more fluid, and they react automatically to their opponent's actions. This aligns with neuroscience findings that flow states occur when the brain's **default mode network**—responsible for daydreaming and self-criticism—becomes less active, allowing athletes to perform at their peak.

### Case Study 3: Flow and Music Performance

Musicians, especially improvisational artists like **jazz players**, frequently experience flow. A study on jazz pianists found that when they were improvising, their brains entered a flow state in which the **lateral prefrontal cortex**—involved in self-monitoring and planning—became less active, allowing the musicians to play freely without overthinking their performance.

**Herbie Hancock**, a renowned jazz pianist, has often spoken about how he enters a state of flow during live performances, where everything else fades away, and he becomes one with the music. Neuroscientists believe this is because flow allows the brain's **reward system** (involving dopamine) to enhance motivation and pleasure, making the experience deeply fulfilling.

## Practical Application

Achieving flow and enhancing focus does not require being a martial artist, musician, or chess player. You can incorporate practical techniques rooted in both neuroscience and ancient wisdom to enhance your cognitive performance in everyday life. Here are some strategies to help you build focus and access flow more regularly:

**Break Tasks into Flow-Friendly Challenges**

To enter flow, your task must be neither too easy nor too difficult. Set clear goals that challenge your current skill level but don't overwhelm you. If a task feels too hard, break it into smaller, more manageable steps. This balance between skill and challenge is vital to reaching flow.

**Limit Distractions**

Flow requires sustained focus, so eliminate distractions before starting a task. Turn off your phone, close unrelated tabs on your computer, and create a quiet workspace. **Environmental triggers**, like music or natural light, can also help set the stage for flow. Neuroscience shows that multitasking prevents deep focus and makes flow impossible, so give your full attention to one task at a time.

**Use Mindfulness to Build Focus**

Integrating mindfulness into your daily routine can strengthen your brain's ability to focus. Spend 5–10 minutes each day practising **mindful breathing** or meditation. Focus on the sensation of your breath, and when distractions arise, gently bring your attention back to your breathing. Over time, this practice will enhance your attention span and make it easier to achieve focus.

**Engage in Rhythmic Activities**

Ancient cultures used rhythmic practices like drumming and chanting to enter flow states. Neuroscientific research shows that rhythmic activities can synchronise brain waves, making focus easier. If you are feeling mentally scattered, try incorporating **walking meditation**, playing an instrument, or rhythmic breathing exercises to realign your focus.

**Physical Movement and Flow**

Incorporate physical activity into your routine, whether through yoga, stretching, or light exercise. Movement not only improves physical health but also primes the brain for flow by increasing **blood flow** and **dopamine levels**. Even short bursts of exercise can reset your brain, helping you re-enter a flow state more easily.

By integrating these techniques into your routine, you can enhance both your cognitive focus and your ability to achieve flow, optimising your performance in personal, creative, and professional endeavours.

## Summary: Enhancing Cognitive Performance with Focus and Ancient Flow States

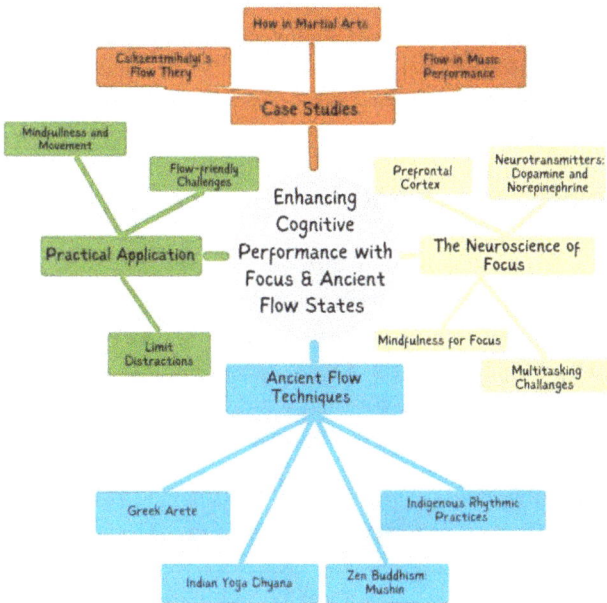

# Chapter 7
# Empathy, Compassion, and the Mirror Neuron System in Ancient Contexts

Empathy and compassion are essential human qualities that foster connection, understanding, and emotional intelligence. Modern neuroscience has provided a deeper understanding of how empathy works, particularly through the discovery of **mirror neurons**—a group of neurons that activate both when we perform an action and when we observe someone else performing the same action. These neurons help us understand others' emotions by simulating their experiences in our own brains. Interestingly, many ancient cultures already had practices in place that cultivated empathy, compassion, and deep social bonds long before the mirror neuron system was understood scientifically.

## Mirror Neurons and Emotional Intelligence

The **mirror neuron system**, discovered in the early 1990s by a team of Italian researchers led by Giacomo Rizzolatti, is a group of neurons in the **premotor cortex** and **inferior parietal lobule** that fire both when a person acts and when they observe someone else performing the same action. This discovery revolutionised our understanding of how we experience empathy and social connection.

When we observe someone experiencing joy, pain, or fear, our mirror neurons activate in a way that allows us to feel a version of that emotion ourselves. For example, when we see someone smile, the same regions in our brain associated with happiness light up, giving us a shared emotional experience. This process helps us understand others' feelings without needing verbal communication, which is why mirror neurons are often considered the foundation of **emotional**

**intelligence**—the ability to perceive, understand, and manage emotions in ourselves and others.

Empathy, driven by the mirror neuron system, plays a crucial role in social bonding, parenting, and cooperative behaviours. **Oxytocin**, often referred to as the "love hormone," is also involved in this process. It reinforces social bonds by fostering feelings of trust and connection. Studies have shown that people with higher levels of emotional intelligence, who can naturally activate these mirror neurons, are better able to navigate social situations and build strong, compassionate relationships.

However, the power of mirror neurons also has a darker side. This system can contribute to **vicarious stress** or **empathy fatigue**, where we become overwhelmed by taking on others' emotions, particularly in high-stress or caregiving roles. This highlights the need for balance between emotional empathy and emotional regulation, both of which are vital components of emotional intelligence.

## Ancient Empathy Practices

Long before neuroscience could explain the biological basis for empathy, ancient cultures developed practices to cultivate compassion and emotional connection within their communities. These practices were integral to maintaining social harmony and strengthening interpersonal bonds, much like how mirror neurons function today.

One prominent example is **Buddhist metta meditation**, also known as **loving-kindness meditation**. This practice involves silently repeating phrases of goodwill toward oneself and others, such as "May you be happy," "May you be healthy," and "May you be free from suffering." Through this meditation, practitioners cultivate a sense of universal empathy and compassion, not just for loved ones but also for strangers and even adversaries. Neuroscientific research supports the efficacy of loving-kindness meditation, showing that it activates brain regions associated with empathy and emotional regulation, such as the **insula** and **anterior cingulate cortex**.

In **ancient Greece**, the philosopher **Aristotle** emphasised the role of empathy (or **phronesis**) in building strong communities. He believed that understanding others' emotions and motivations was crucial for ethical behaviour and maintaining social harmony. The **Greek concept of "catharsis"**—the emotional release experienced through art, particularly theatre—also highlights the ancient understanding of empathy. Greek tragedies were designed to evoke deep emotional reactions from audiences, fostering a collective sense of compassion and shared experience.

**Indigenous cultures** across the globe also placed high importance on empathy, particularly in **oral traditions** where storytelling was used to convey collective experiences. For example, in many African communities, storytelling was a tool for teaching moral lessons, encouraging listeners to step into the shoes of others. This practice not only transmitted cultural values but also nurtured empathy and social cohesion.

In **Hinduism**, the principle of **Ahimsa**—non-violence—is rooted in empathy and compassion. Ahimsa extends beyond physical actions to include thoughts and intentions, encouraging people to consider the emotional and psychological impact of their actions on others. This principle resonates with the modern understanding of emotional intelligence, as it promotes thoughtful consideration of others' emotions and well-being.

These ancient empathy practices, though varied across cultures, share a common goal: fostering deep emotional connections, compassion, and mutual understanding, which are as vital in modern societies as they were in ancient ones.

## Case Studies

### Case Study 1: Mirror Neurons and Autism Spectrum Disorder (ASD)

Autism Spectrum Disorder (ASD) is often associated with difficulties in social interaction and empathy. Neuroscientists have hypothesised that individuals with ASD may have impairments in their mirror neuron systems, which could explain some of the challenges they face in understanding and mimicking others' emotions. While research is ongoing, several studies suggest that the mirror neuron system functions differently in people with ASD, particularly in regions responsible for processing social cues.

One groundbreaking study used **fMRI** to observe the brains of children with ASD while they watched facial expressions of different emotions. The study found reduced activation in critical areas of the mirror neuron system, such as the **inferior frontal gyrus**. Despite these challenges, therapies that focus on increasing social engagement and emotional recognition, such as **social skills training** and **empathy-building exercises**, have been shown to improve emotional intelligence in individuals with ASD.

### Case Study 2: Buddhist Monks and Compassion Training

Neuroscientific research on Buddhist monks who have spent decades practising **loving-kindness meditation** reveals fascinating insights into how empathy can be trained and enhanced. One study, led by **Dr Richard Davidson** at the University of Wisconsin, scanned the brains of Tibetan monks who practised compassion meditation for years. The results showed increased activity in the **insula** and **temporal parietal junction**—brain regions involved in empathy and emotional understanding.

Interestingly, the monks were able to generate intense feelings of compassion not only for loved ones but for all living beings, including those who had wronged them. This suggests that empathy, like many other cognitive abilities, can be enhanced through intentional practice, offering hope for therapies aimed at increasing emotional intelligence in broader populations.

### Case Study 3: Mirror Neurons in Leadership and Corporate Empathy

A CEO of a large tech company dealing with high employee turnover decided to implement empathy training within the organisation. The training focused on enhancing emotional intelligence among managers, encouraging them to practise active listening and perspective-taking, core skills associated with the mirror neuron system. Over time, the company saw improvements in employee satisfaction, productivity, and retention.

Neuroscientific studies support this approach, showing that leaders who practice empathy and compassion are more likely to foster trust and loyalty among their teams. Mirror neurons are thought to be critical in leadership because they help leaders intuitively understand the emotional needs of their employees, allowing for better communication and more effective conflict resolution.

# Practical Tips

Cultivating empathy and compassion can be a transformative practice, not only for improving personal relationships but also for enhancing professional and social interactions. Here are practical strategies, grounded in both neuroscience and ancient wisdom, for enhancing empathy and emotional intelligence:

### Practice Loving-Kindness Meditation

Set aside 10–15 minutes a day to practise loving-kindness meditation, similar to the Buddhist practice of metta. Begin by sending kind thoughts to yourself, then expand to others—family, friends, colleagues, and eventually, even difficult people in your life. Research shows that regular practice can strengthen the neural circuits responsible for empathy and compassion.

### Engage in Active Listening

Mirror neurons are activated when we truly listen to others. The next time you are in a conversation, focus entirely on the speaker—make eye contact, nod to show understanding, and avoid interrupting. Active listening helps you feel the other person's emotions and respond with empathy.

## Use Empathy Mapping

This technique, often used in design thinking, helps you step into someone else's shoes. To use an empathy map, write down what the person you are focusing on might be thinking, feeling, seeing, and doing in a given situation. This simple exercise strengthens your ability to understand others' emotions and perspectives.

## Reduce Empathy Fatigue

If you find yourself overwhelmed by others' emotions—especially in caregiving or high-stress professions—practice self-care to maintain a healthy balance between empathy and emotional regulation. Techniques like mindfulness, setting boundaries, and regularly engaging in activities that recharge your energy can prevent empathy fatigue.

## Empathy Journaling

Keep a daily journal where you reflect on moments when you felt empathy or compassion for others. Write about what triggered these feelings and how you responded. Over time, this practice will enhance your emotional intelligence and make empathy a more automatic response in daily interactions.

By integrating these practices into your routine, you can enhance your empathy and emotional intelligence, fostering deeper, more meaningful connections with others while also improving your ability to navigate social and professional environments.

# Summary: Empathy, Compassion, and the Mirror Neuron System in Ancient Contexts

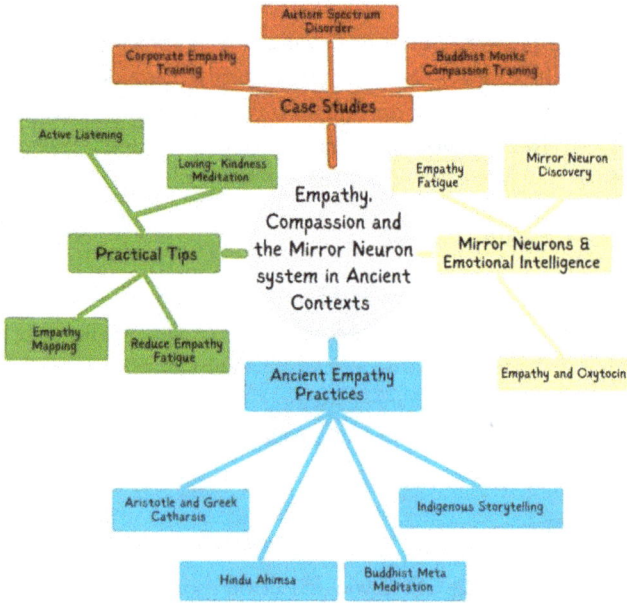

# Chapter 8
# Leadership, Influence, and Ancient Philosophical Approaches

## Brain Chemistry of Leadership

Leadership is not just about charisma or decision-making skills; it is also deeply connected to brain chemistry. Neuroscience has identified key neurotransmitters and brain regions that influence how leaders make decisions, manage stress, and inspire others. Understanding the **brain chemistry of leadership** provides insight into why some people are naturally inclined toward leadership roles and how others can develop these skills.

One of the most important chemicals in leadership is **dopamine**, often referred to as the "motivation molecule." Dopamine is linked to the brain's reward system and plays a critical role in motivation, goal-setting, and risk-taking. Leaders often have higher baseline levels of dopamine, which can drive them to pursue goals with focus and determination. Dopamine also encourages creativity and innovation, traits often associated with visionary leadership.

Another critical hormone is **oxytocin**, sometimes called the "bonding hormone." Oxytocin strengthens social bonds and trust, which is essential for effective leadership. Leaders who can foster a sense of trust and loyalty within their teams tend to be more successful, and oxytocin is at the heart of this process. High oxytocin levels make leaders appear more empathetic, compassionate, and approachable, helping them build stronger relationships with those they lead.

In contrast, **cortisol**, the stress hormone, can undermine leadership if not properly managed. Elevated cortisol levels over prolonged periods can lead to poor decision-making, emotional volatility, and burnout. The ability to manage stress effectively—keeping cortisol in check—is crucial for maintaining long-term leadership success. Leaders who practice mindfulness, meditation, or physical activity tend to have better control over their cortisol levels, allowing them to stay calm under pressure.

**Serotonin** also plays a significant role in leadership. This neurotransmitter regulates mood, emotional stability, and social dominance. High serotonin levels contribute to a sense of confidence and well-being, traits that are essential in leadership. Leaders who exhibit calm, rational thinking even in the face of challenges are often those with balanced serotonin levels.

The **prefrontal cortex** is the brain region responsible for higher-order thinking, planning, and emotional regulation—crucial skills for any leader. It helps in evaluating complex situations, managing impulses, and making well-informed decisions. Effective leaders often have highly active prefrontal cortices, enabling them to remain composed and rational, even in high-stress situations.

By understanding the role of these neurotransmitters and brain regions, we can begin to see why certain individuals excel in leadership roles and how others can develop the necessary skills to lead effectively. The chemistry of the brain, when balanced and nurtured, supports the qualities we associate with strong, resilient leadership.

## Ancient Leadership Philosophies

Long before neuroscience could explain the brain chemistry behind leadership, ancient civilisations developed philosophical frameworks to understand what makes a great leader. These philosophies, many of which remain influential today, offer timeless insights into leadership qualities such as wisdom, empathy, courage, and justice.

In **ancient Greece**, **Plato** and **Aristotle** both explored the concept of leadership through the lens of virtue. Plato, in his work *The Republic*, described the ideal leader as a philosopher-king—a ruler guided by wisdom and reason rather than personal ambition or emotional impulses. According to Plato, the philosopher-king is uniquely equipped to lead because of their commitment to truth, justice, and the greater good. This idea resonates with modern notions of servant leadership, where leaders prioritise the well-being of their team or community over personal gain.

**Aristotle**, on the other hand, emphasised the importance of **ethical leadership**. In his work *Politics*, Aristotle argued that a good leader must possess practical wisdom, or **phronesis**—the ability to make sound judgments in the face of uncertainty. He also stressed the importance of **empathy** and understanding the needs of the people. Aristotle believed that leaders should cultivate virtues such as courage, temperance, and justice, as these traits would help them balance their personal desires with the needs of the broader society.

In **ancient China**, **Confucius** outlined a philosophy of leadership based on moral integrity and benevolence. Confucius believed that the foundation of leadership was **virtue (de)**, and that a leader must lead by example. The concept of **ren**, or humaneness, was central to Confucian leadership philosophy. Confucius argued that leaders must exhibit compassion, fairness, and respect for others. When leaders act with virtue and integrity, they naturally inspire loyalty and trust within their followers. This is similar to the modern understanding of leadership based on emotional intelligence and the importance of building trust within teams.

**Sun Tzu**, another influential Chinese thinker, approached leadership from a strategic perspective in his work *The Art of War*. He emphasised the importance of **adaptability**, **strategic thinking**, and understanding both the strengths and weaknesses of one's followers and enemies. Sun Tzu's philosophy of leadership involved knowing when to act and when to remain patient, and how to inspire confidence without unnecessary conflict. His ideas are often applied in modern business leadership, where the ability to navigate complex and competitive environments is crucial.

In **ancient India**, the text of the **Bhagavad Gita** offers a philosophical framework for leadership that blends duty, courage, and selflessness. The warrior Arjuna is guided by Lord Krishna to understand that leadership is not about personal victory but about fulfilling one's duty to others with integrity and dedication. This aligns with the modern idea of purpose-driven leadership, where leaders are motivated by a sense of service to a larger cause rather than personal gain.

These ancient philosophies provide a foundation for leadership that transcends time. They emphasise the importance of wisdom, moral integrity, empathy, and strategic thinking—qualities that are as essential today as they were thousands of years ago.

## Case Studies

### Case Study 1: Modern Leadership and Dopamine-Driven Motivation

One example of how dopamine impacts leadership is seen in **Elon Musk**, the CEO of Tesla and SpaceX. Musk's relentless drive to innovate and achieve ambitious goals is often cited as a defining feature of his leadership style. His dopamine-driven motivation allows him to take risks and push the boundaries of technology, from developing electric cars to launching rockets into space. Musk's willingness to take on seemingly impossible projects, despite the odds, reflects high levels of dopamine, which fuels his capacity for innovation and goal setting.

However, this kind of dopamine-driven leadership can also lead to burnout or poor decision-making if not balanced with emotional regulation and stress management. Musk has openly admitted to experiencing stress and sleep deprivation, highlighting the need for leaders to balance dopamine-fueled ambition with practices that support mental and emotional well-being.

### Case Study 2: Empathy in Leadership - Jacinda Ardern

New Zealand's Prime Minister, **Jacinda Ardern,** is often praised for her empathetic leadership style, particularly in times of crisis. Following the 2019 Christchurch mosque shootings, Ardern's immediate response was one of compassion, unity, and empathy. She met with the victims' families, addressed the nation with a message of inclusivity, and wore a hijab as a sign of respect for the Muslim community. Her actions demonstrated a high level of emotional intelligence and the ability to connect deeply with her people.

Ardern's leadership style is an example of how **oxytocin**, the bonding hormone, can be at the heart of effective leadership. By fostering trust and emotional connection, Ardern was able to unite her country in the aftermath of tragedy, showing that empathy is a powerful tool for leadership in both politics and business.

### Case Study 3: Leadership Stress and Cortisol Management - Tim Cook

As the CEO of Apple, **Tim Cook** leads one of the most influential companies in the world. While the pressure of running such a massive organisation could easily lead to burnout, Cook is known for his ability to manage stress effectively. His daily routine includes waking up at 4:00 AM to exercise, a practice that helps him manage his cortisol levels and start the day with mental clarity.

Cook's approach to leadership highlights the importance of balancing high-pressure decision-making with stress management practices. By maintaining a routine that keeps his cortisol levels in check, Cook is able to perform at a high level without sacrificing his mental and emotional well-being.

## Practical Application

Leaders can enhance their performance and well-being by applying insights from neuroscience and ancient wisdom to their leadership styles. Here are some practical strategies for developing leadership skills based on brain chemistry and timeless philosophical principles:

**Boost Dopamine with Goal-Setting and Rewards**

Dopamine is the neurotransmitter that drives motivation and ambition. To harness this, break larger goals into smaller, achievable tasks. Celebrating small wins triggers dopamine release, keeping you motivated throughout the process. Leaders can use this technique to maintain focus and drive in themselves and their teams.

**Build Trust and Compassion with Oxytocin**

Empathy and trust are crucial for leadership. To foster a sense of connection within your team, practice active listening, show appreciation, and encourage collaboration. Regularly checking in with team members and recognising their contributions can stimulate oxytocin, reinforcing positive social bonds.

**Manage Stress with Cortisol-Reducing Practices**

To prevent burnout and maintain emotional stability, incorporate stress-reducing practices into your routine. Techniques such as mindfulness meditation, regular physical exercise, and deep breathing exercises can help keep cortisol levels in check, allowing leaders to stay calm and focused under pressure.

**Incorporate Ancient Leadership Wisdom**

Draw from ancient philosophies that emphasise ethical and empathetic leadership. Practice **self-reflection** as recommended by Confucius, engage in **strategic thinking** like Sun Tzu, and cultivate **virtue-based leadership** as outlined by Aristotle. These practices encourage leaders to act with integrity, build stronger relationships, and make better decisions in complex situations.

**Foster Emotional Intelligence**

Work on developing your emotional intelligence by understanding the role of mirror neurons. By increasing your awareness of how others feel and practising empathy, you can improve your ability to lead with compassion and connect on a deeper level with your team.

## Summary: Leadership, Influence, and Ancient Philosophical Approaches

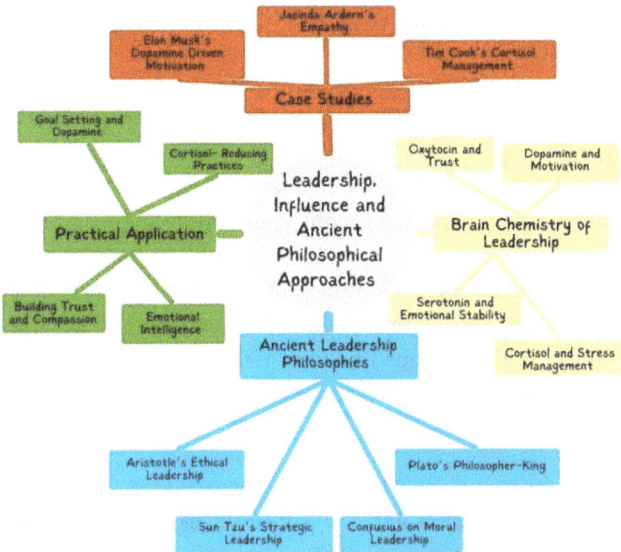

# Chapter 9
# The Brain-Body Connection
# and Ancient Holistic Health

## The Brain-Body Connection

The **brain-body connection** is one of the most fascinating and well-researched areas in modern neuroscience. The brain communicates with every part of the body through a vast network of nerves, hormones, and chemicals, allowing for the integration of physical and mental health. The **central nervous system (CNS)**, consisting of the brain and spinal cord, controls voluntary movements, sensory information, and reflexes. It also regulates involuntary processes like breathing, heartbeat, digestion, and even immune responses through the **autonomic nervous system (ANS)**, which includes the sympathetic ("fight or flight") and parasympathetic ("rest and digest") systems.

In recent years, the brain-body connection has been further illuminated by research into the **gut-brain axis**, a communication network between the gut microbiome and the brain. Gut health, influenced by diet, stress, and lifestyle, directly impacts mood, cognition, and overall mental health through pathways involving the vagus nerve and the production of neurotransmitters like **serotonin**, 90% of which is produced in the gut. This connection illustrates how our physical health influences emotional and cognitive well-being, as well as how mental states can affect bodily functions such as immune responses, metabolism, and cardiovascular health.

The **hypothalamus**, a small but powerful region of the brain, plays a crucial role in regulating the brain-body connection by managing hormones, including **cortisol** (stress hormone), **adrenaline**, and **oxytocin** (bonding hormone). These chemicals influence not just how we feel but how our bodies respond to external stimuli, such as stress, danger, or pleasure. Chronic stress, for example, can lead to sustained high cortisol levels, which are linked to cardiovascular problems, weakened immune function, and mental health disorders like anxiety and depression.

Understanding the intricate brain-body connection has led to innovative approaches in treating conditions like chronic pain, stress-related disorders, and autoimmune diseases. It also reinforces the importance of maintaining physical health through lifestyle factors like diet, exercise, and sleep to support mental clarity and emotional resilience.

## Ancient Holistic Practices

Long before neuroscience illuminated the brain-body connection, **ancient cultures** recognised the intricate link between mental, physical, and spiritual health. Ancient holistic practices, though lacking the scientific framework we have today, were based on the intuitive understanding that the mind and body are deeply interconnected. These practices aimed to maintain harmony between the mind, body, and spirit, promoting long-term health and well-being.

**Ayurveda**, a 5,000-year-old system of medicine from India, is one of the most comprehensive examples of ancient holistic health. Central to Ayurveda is the idea of **balance**, specifically between the three **doshas**—Vata (air and space), Pitta (fire and water), and Kapha (earth and water). Each person has a unique combination of these doshas. When they fall out of balance, it can lead to physical and mental illness. Ayurveda emphasises the use of diet, herbal treatments, yoga, and meditation to bring the mind and body into balance, echoing modern understandings of the gut-brain axis and the importance of lifestyle in maintaining brain health.

In **Traditional Chinese Medicine (TCM)**, the concept of **Qi** (life force) governs all health practices. TCM views the body as a system of interconnected organs, much like how modern neuroscience views the body as interconnected with the brain. Practices such as **acupuncture** and **Tai Chi** work to regulate the flow of Qi, ensuring balance between the body's energies. Modern research supports acupuncture's ability to reduce pain by stimulating nerves, muscles, and connective tissues, as well as its effect on activating the brain's natural painkillers—endorphins.

**Hippocratic medicine**, originating in ancient Greece, emphasised the importance of diet, exercise, and mental balance. Hippocrates believed that the health of the body directly influenced the health of the mind and vice versa. His focus on prevention through a healthy lifestyle has strong parallels with modern preventive medicine and neuroscience, which advocates for the benefits of a healthy diet, regular physical activity, and stress management techniques like mindfulness for maintaining cognitive and emotional well-being.

Another ancient practice that recognised the brain-body connection is **yoga**, which combines physical postures, breath control, and meditation. Yoga's focus on **pranayama** (breath control) directly links to modern understandings of how breath affects the autonomic nervous system. Deep, controlled breathing stimulates the parasympathetic nervous system, reducing stress and calming the mind—scientifically validated as reducing cortisol and improving focus and mental clarity.

By combining movement, mindfulness, and balanced living, these ancient holistic practices offer timeless strategies for optimising both physical and mental health. The growing body of scientific research supports many of the principles these practices advocated, confirming that maintaining balance in the body can lead to mental resilience and cognitive sharpness.

# Case Studies

### Case Study 1: Chronic Pain Management through Mind-Body Practices

Jane, a 45-year-old teacher, had suffered from chronic lower back pain for over a decade. Despite trying various treatments, including medication and physical therapy, her pain persisted. Frustrated, she turned to holistic practices, combining modern neuroscience and ancient techniques like **yoga** and **meditation**. Yoga helped Jane build core strength, improve posture, and increase flexibility, all of which reduced the physical stress on her spine. Simultaneously, practising mindfulness meditation allowed her to shift her focus away from the pain, reducing its psychological impact. Over time, her pain decreased significantly, and she felt more in control of her body.

Scientific studies show that **mindfulness meditation** and **yoga** can reduce pain by altering the way the brain perceives it. Brain scans of chronic pain sufferers practising mindfulness show decreased activity in the **amygdala** (responsible for pain perception) and increased connectivity in the **prefrontal cortex** (involved in cognitive control). Jane's case highlights how ancient practices can complement modern treatments by targeting both the mental and physical aspects of chronic pain.

**Case Study 2: Stress Management through Ayurveda**

Arjun, a 35-year-old engineer, struggled with chronic stress and anxiety. Conventional treatments, including medication, provided only temporary relief. He decided to explore **Ayurveda**, seeking balance through personalised dietary recommendations, herbal supplements, and **pranayama** (breathing exercises). Under the guidance of an Ayurvedic practitioner, Arjun adjusted his diet to reduce his Pitta dosha, which Ayurveda associates with heat, stress, and inflammation. He also practised pranayama daily, calming his mind and improving his focus.

After several months, Arjun reported significantly lower stress levels and improved mental clarity. His cortisol levels, measured before and after the intervention, had decreased by 20%. Modern research supports these findings: **breath control** techniques like pranayama activate the parasympathetic nervous system, reducing cortisol production and improving stress resilience.

### Case Study 3: Gut-Brain Health through Traditional Chinese Medicine

Sophia, a 50-year-old marketing executive, struggled with irritable bowel syndrome (IBS), which worsened her anxiety and affected her cognitive performance. After reading about the **gut-brain axis**, she sought help from a practitioner of **Traditional Chinese Medicine (TCM)**. Sophia began acupuncture sessions, along with dietary changes to balance her Qi. Acupuncture targeted specific points to reduce anxiety and regulate digestion, while the diet aimed to soothe inflammation in her gut.

After 12 weeks, Sophia's IBS symptoms had improved, and she reported feeling less anxious and more mentally focused. Research shows that acupuncture can reduce inflammation, stimulate the release of serotonin, and regulate gut motility, thus supporting both gut and brain health.

## Practical Tips

To strengthen the brain-body connection and promote overall well-being, consider these practical tips inspired by ancient holistic practices and supported by modern neuroscience:

### Practice Mindful Movement

Engage in practices like yoga, Tai Chi, or even simple stretching. These activities enhance both physical flexibility and mental clarity. By combining movement with mindful breathing, you activate the parasympathetic nervous system, reducing stress hormones like cortisol and promoting relaxation. Studies show that even moderate exercise increases neuroplasticity, boosting brain health.

## Incorporate Breathwork

Breathing exercises, like pranayama or deep diaphragmatic breathing, can help regulate the autonomic nervous system. By practising deep, controlled breathing, you can shift from the "fight or flight" sympathetic response to the "rest and digest" parasympathetic state. Try spending five minutes each day focusing on slow, deep breaths to lower stress and increase focus.

## Optimise Gut Health for Brain Health

Focus on a diet that promotes gut health, rich in fibre, probiotics, and anti-inflammatory foods. The gut-brain axis plays a crucial role in mental health, so supporting the gut microbiome can reduce anxiety and improve cognitive function. Foods like fermented vegetables, yoghurt, and whole grains can support the gut and, in turn, the brain.

## Adopt a Balanced Lifestyle

Inspired by Ayurveda and other holistic systems, aim for balance in your diet, sleep, and work life. Regular sleep patterns, a nutritious diet, and physical activity all support the brain-body connection. Modern neuroscience validates that consistency in these areas improves cognitive performance and emotional resilience.

## Incorporate Meditation and Mindfulness

Take time each day to meditate or practice mindfulness. These techniques enhance focus, reduce anxiety, and foster resilience. Meditation strengthens the **prefrontal cortex**, the brain region responsible for executive functions like decision-making and emotional control, which can help you manage stress more effectively.

# Summary: The Brain-Body Connection and Ancient Holistic Health

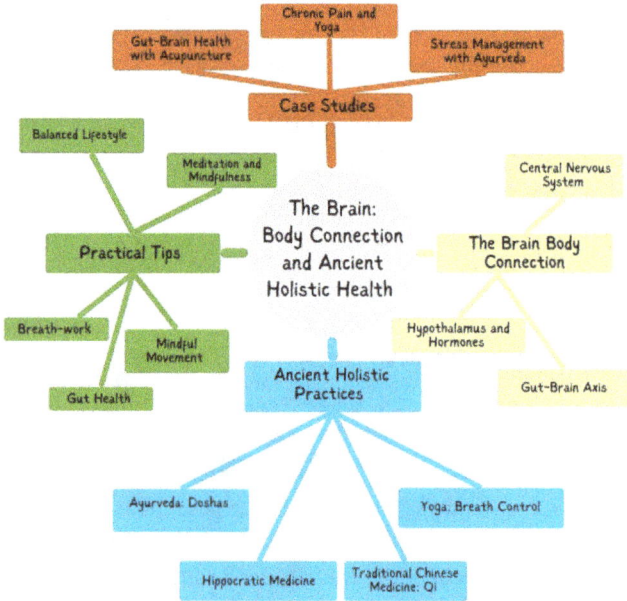

# Chapter 10
# Pain Perception and Ancient Pain Management Techniques

## The Neuroscience of Chronic Pain

Chronic pain is a condition where pain signals continue to be sent to the brain even after the initial injury or source of pain has healed. This persistent pain is a result of changes in the brain and nervous system, where pain pathways become overactive and the brain becomes hypersensitive to pain signals. Understanding how chronic pain works in the brain is essential to finding effective ways to manage it.

The **nociceptors**, or pain receptors, detect injury and send signals to the brain through the spinal cord. In cases of chronic pain, however, the nervous system becomes "rewired" in a process called **central sensitisation**. This rewiring leads to a heightened sensitivity to pain. It can make non-painful stimuli (like a light touch) feel painful. The **amygdala**, responsible for emotional processing, and the **anterior cingulate cortex**, involved in the emotional response to pain, also become more active in chronic pain, linking the sensation of pain to emotional suffering.

Chronic pain can also lead to changes in the brain's **grey matter**, particularly in regions like the **prefrontal cortex**, which controls decision-making and emotional regulation, and the **thalamus**, the relay centre for sensory signals. These changes not only make the pain feel more intense but also affect mood, attention, and cognitive function.

Modern neuroscience has also revealed the critical role of **neuroinflammation** in chronic pain. Prolonged pain can lead to inflammation in the nervous system, which can sustain the pain cycle. Additionally, stress plays a crucial role in exacerbating chronic pain through the release of **cortisol**, which can heighten pain sensitivity.

In response to chronic pain, treatments often aim to "retrain" the brain and nervous system to reduce the hypersensitivity and emotional responses associated with pain. This neuroplasticity-based approach shows that the brain, even in chronic pain, can change, heal, and adapt, much like it does in other conditions that involve nervous system rewiring.

## Ancient Pain Management

Ancient cultures, long before the advent of modern medicine, developed various pain management techniques that focused on the mind-body connection. Many of these techniques align with contemporary understandings of the neuroscience of pain, emphasising the importance of altering the perception of pain rather than just eliminating it.

One of the most well-known ancient pain management techniques is **acupuncture**, which originated in **Traditional Chinese Medicine (TCM)** over 2,500 years ago. Acupuncture involves inserting thin needles into specific points on the body to balance the flow of **Qi**, or energy, and promote healing. From a modern perspective, acupuncture is believed to stimulate the nervous system, triggering the release of pain-relieving chemicals like **endorphins** and **serotonin**. Research has shown that acupuncture can help modulate pain signals in the brain by affecting areas such as the **thalamus**, **amygdala**, and **hypothalamus**, reducing the perception of pain.

In **Ayurvedic medicine**, pain was often treated through the use of herbal remedies, massage, and **pranayama** (breath control). For example, herbs like **turmeric** and **ginger** have long been used for their anti-inflammatory properties, reducing pain and swelling. Ayurveda also emphasises the balancing of the body's energy systems (the doshas), which can lead to improved pain tolerance. Practices like pranayama help to regulate the nervous system and reduce stress, which is now understood to play a significant role in managing chronic pain.

In ancient **Egypt,** pain relief methods included the use of natural analgesics like **willow bark,** which contains **salicylic acid,** the active ingredient in aspirin. Egyptian healers also used massage and prayer to treat pain, recognising the importance of the emotional and spiritual aspects of healing.

The **Greeks and Romans** were also advanced in their understanding of pain management. **Hippocrates** recommended hydrotherapy (water therapy) and natural remedies like opium and vinegar for pain relief. Roman physicians like **Galen** used opium for its potent analgesic effects while also emphasising exercise and a balanced diet as essential components of overall health, which in turn reduced pain.

These ancient practices show that managing pain has long been understood as a holistic process involving both the mind and body. Techniques that reduce stress, improve emotional well-being, and focus on altering the perception of pain have stood the test of time, and many are still used in combination with modern medical treatments today.

## Case Studies

### Case Study 1: Acupuncture for Chronic Migraine Relief

Laura, a 37-year-old marketing professional, had suffered from debilitating migraines for over a decade. After trying multiple medications with little success, she turned to acupuncture based on a recommendation from a colleague. Over the course of three months, Laura received weekly acupuncture treatments that targeted specific points known to relieve migraine pain, such as the **LI4 (Hegu)** and **GB20 (Fengchi)** points.

After 12 sessions, Laura reported a significant reduction in the frequency and intensity of her migraines. Brain imaging studies of acupuncture patients have shown reduced activity in the **cingulate gyrus**, the area of the brain associated with the emotional experience of pain, and increased activation in the prefrontal cortex, which is responsible for pain modulation. Laura's experience demonstrates how an ancient technique like acupuncture can effectively manage chronic pain by altering the brain's pain pathways.

### Case Study 2: Ayurvedic Pranayama for Fibromyalgia

James, a 50-year-old teacher, struggled with **fibromyalgia**. This chronic pain condition affects muscles and soft tissues, causing widespread pain and fatigue. Seeking relief, James incorporated Ayurvedic breathing techniques, specifically **pranayama**, into his daily routine. By focusing on deep diaphragmatic breathing and alternating nostril breathing, he was able to reduce his pain perception and anxiety levels.

Pranayama helped James stimulate the parasympathetic nervous system, reducing the body's stress response and promoting relaxation. This practice aligned with his treatment plan, which also included physical therapy and a balanced diet. Research on pranayama and fibromyalgia shows that these breathing techniques can reduce stress hormones like cortisol, which often exacerbate chronic pain. Over several months, James experienced significant improvement in both pain levels and overall well-being.

### Case Study 3: Meditation for Chronic Back Pain

Sophie, a 42-year-old office worker, had been living with chronic lower back pain for five years. After conventional treatments failed, she turned to **mindfulness-based stress reduction (MBSR)**, a technique rooted in ancient meditation practices. By practising mindfulness meditation for 30 minutes a day, Sophie learned to focus on her breath and observe her pain without reacting emotionally to it.

Mindfulness has been shown to change the way the brain perceives pain by reducing activity in the **default mode network (DMN)** and the amygdala, areas involved in the emotional response to pain. Within six months, Sophie reported feeling more in control of her pain and less emotionally distressed by it. Her pain had not disappeared entirely, but her ability to manage it had dramatically improved, allowing her to return to normal activities with minimal discomfort.

## Practical Application

Ancient pain management techniques offer valuable insights into how we can approach chronic pain holistically, combining mind-body practices with modern science. Here are practical steps to apply these methods in everyday life:

### Incorporate Acupuncture

Consider exploring acupuncture if you suffer from chronic pain conditions like migraines, arthritis, or fibromyalgia. Research a qualified practitioner and aim for a series of sessions, as results often improve over time. The practice can help release endorphins and regulate pain signals in the brain, offering a non-invasive, drug-free option for pain relief.

### Practice Mindfulness Meditation

Mindfulness meditation, rooted in ancient Buddhist practices, is an effective tool for managing chronic pain by shifting your relationship to it. Spend 10-15 minutes each day practising mindfulness. Focus on your breath or a specific part of your body, and observe your thoughts without judgment. Over time, this practice can help reduce the emotional distress associated with chronic pain, making it more manageable.

### Use Breathwork Techniques (Pranayama)

Breathing exercises, such as pranayama, can help alleviate chronic pain by stimulating the parasympathetic nervous system, which reduces the body's stress response. Try practising **alternate nostril breathing** or deep diaphragmatic breathing for 5-10 minutes each day. This practice can reduce cortisol levels, improve emotional resilience, and lower pain perception.

**Herbal Remedies**

Incorporate natural anti-inflammatory herbs like **turmeric, ginger**, and **willow bark** into your diet or as supplements. These herbs have been used for centuries to manage pain and inflammation, and modern research supports their effectiveness in reducing pain in conditions like arthritis and chronic joint pain.

**Regular Movement**

While chronic pain often makes movement difficult, gentle exercises like **yoga** or **Tai Chi** can help improve mobility and reduce pain. These mind-body practices increase flexibility, strengthen muscles, and promote relaxation, which can alleviate pain over time. Start with small, manageable routines and gradually increase your activity level as your pain subsides.

By combining ancient wisdom with modern neuroscience, you can take a proactive approach to managing chronic pain in ways that align both the mind and body. These holistic techniques provide sustainable, long-term strategies for reducing pain and enhancing overall well-being.

# Summary: Pain Perception and Ancient Pain Management Techniques

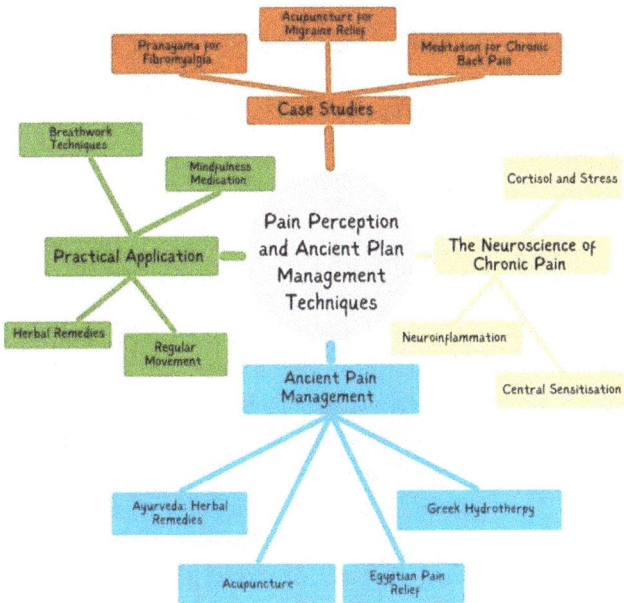

# Chapter 11
# Brain-Computer Interfaces and Neurotechnology Aligned with Ancient Philosophies

## Neuroscience and AI

The rapid advancement of neuroscience and artificial intelligence (AI) is redefining the boundaries of human capability. Brain-computer interfaces (BCIs) and neurotechnology enable a direct link between the brain and external devices, allowing individuals to control machines, communicate, and even restore lost functions using their thoughts. This revolutionary technology taps into our brain's electrical signals, translating them into actionable commands that can move robotic limbs, type on a computer, or control prosthetic devices.

Neuroscientific research has revealed that the brain operates through intricate networks of neurons that communicate via electrical impulses. BCIs harness this electrical activity, particularly in regions like the motor cortex, which is responsible for movement. For instance, stroke survivors or those with paralysis can learn to use BCIs to control a robotic arm by simply thinking about moving their own arm. This convergence of AI and neuroscience promises to restore mobility, independence, and even communication to those with neurological impairments.

Advancements in AI also play a critical role in improving the functionality of BCIs. Machine learning algorithms can be trained to interpret brain signals more accurately, allowing for seamless interaction between the brain and machines. This has implications beyond healthcare, including applications in gaming, education, and personal productivity, where BCIs can enhance human-computer interaction.

However, as we enhance our cognitive and physical capabilities with technology, ethical questions arise about the nature of human identity, free will, and privacy. As BCIs move from laboratories into everyday use, we must consider how these technologies align with our evolving understanding of what it means to be human.

## Ancient Mind-Body Connection

While BCIs and neurotechnology represent the forefront of modern scientific advancement, the core concept of connecting the mind and body is deeply rooted in ancient philosophies. Cultures around the world, from ancient Egypt to Greece and India, have long acknowledged the inseparable link between the mind and body in health, cognition, and personal mastery.

In ancient India, the concept of "prana" (life force) flows through the body and mind, connecting mental and physical states. Yoga, meditation, and Ayurvedic practices were built around cultivating harmony between mind and body, emphasising breath control, physical postures, and focused attention to optimise well-being. Modern neuroscience has confirmed that these practices positively affect brain function, from enhancing focus to improving emotional regulation by engaging areas of the brain like the prefrontal cortex and reducing activity in the amygdala, which governs the fear response.

Similarly, in ancient Greece, philosophers like Plato and Aristotle recognised the importance of the mind-body connection. Aristotle's theory of "hylomorphism" proposed that the mind and body are deeply interconnected, each influencing the other in profound ways. Plato's "tri-partite" theory of the soul placed reason (mind), spirit, and physical desires in a delicate balance to achieve a life of virtue. Modern neurotechnology, particularly BCIs, echoes this ancient understanding by physically linking brain activity with external tools, thus manifesting thought into action.

These ancient perspectives remind us that as we advance technologically, we must maintain a balance between technological enhancement and our inherent biological wisdom. The goal of using BCIs should not only be to expand physical capacities but also to deepen the connection between mind, body, and technology holistically.

## Case Studies

One remarkable case is that of Jan Scheuermann, a woman who became quadriplegic due to a rare genetic disorder. Through BCI technology, she was able to control a robotic arm using only her thoughts. By linking her brain activity to the mechanical arm, she performed complex movements, such as shaking hands and feeding herself—tasks she hadn't been able to do in years. This was possible due to electrodes implanted in her motor cortex, which communicated with the robotic arm in real-time, demonstrating how BCIs can restore a sense of autonomy.

Another example is that of ALS (Amyotrophic Lateral Sclerosis) patients who, having lost their ability to speak or move, have used BCIs to communicate again. In these cases, non-invasive BCIs that use electroencephalography (EEG) sensors placed on the scalp detect brain waves and allow patients to spell out words on a screen by simply focusing on individual letters. This ability to re-establish communication via brain signals has not only improved quality of life but has also reaffirmed their sense of agency.

In the realm of gaming, BCIs are beginning to revolutionise the way individuals interact with virtual environments. Neuro-gaming companies are exploring how players can control avatars, manipulate objects, or engage in strategic gameplay using brainwaves. This level of immersion, controlled solely by thought, represents a new frontier of interactive entertainment that connects mind and machine on a deeper level.

These cases illustrate how BCIs have already begun transforming lives by reconnecting the mind with actions once thought lost.

Whether in healthcare or entertainment, the implications of BCIs are profound, opening doors to both restoration and enhancement of human capability.

## Practical Application

The practical applications of BCIs and neurotechnology offer exciting possibilities for personal and professional development. Here's how you can start engaging with the emerging world of neurotechnology and mind-body integration:

### Brain Training through Neurofeedback

Neurofeedback systems, available in devices like the Muse headband or Emotiv's EEG headsets, offer a form of non-invasive neurotechnology. These devices monitor brainwaves and provide feedback to help users optimise focus, relaxation, or creativity. Whether you are seeking better concentration at work or improved meditation practices, neurofeedback trains your brain to regulate itself, enhancing mental performance. The feedback loop created between brain activity and external sensors enables users to strengthen cognitive control, much like physical training strengthens muscles.

### Meditation and Mindfulness with Neurotechnology

Many ancient mind-body techniques, such as meditation and yoga, are now supported by neurotech devices. You can use neurofeedback during meditation sessions to track and improve your brain's relaxation state in real-time. Mindfulness apps combined with EEG sensors can help deepen your practice, merging ancient wisdom with modern technological enhancement for a more profound connection between mind and body.

**Enhancing Physical Rehabilitation**

BCIs offer new opportunities for physical rehabilitation by encouraging neuroplasticity. Those recovering from injury or illness, such as stroke patients or individuals with motor impairments, can incorporate brain-controlled devices into their therapy to regain function. You can explore partnerships with medical professionals specialising in neurorehabilitation to utilise BCI-assisted therapy, blending traditional physical therapy with cutting-edge neurotechnology.

**Cognitive Enhancement for Focus and Creativity**

In both professional and creative fields, BCIs offer tools to enhance cognitive performance. Developers and tech enthusiasts can explore BCI-integrated tools to boost concentration, solve problems faster, or unlock new levels of creativity. Devices like FocusBand, which tracks brainwaves to optimise attention, offer the practical benefits of improved workflow and higher productivity.

Ultimately, the practical applications of BCIs are not just about improving physical abilities but also about deepening the integration of our mind, body, and technology. Combining the wisdom of ancient mind-body techniques with the future of neurotechnology allows us to expand human potential and redefine what it means to be truly connected in the modern world.

# Summary: Brain-Computer Interfaces and Neurotechnology Aligned with Ancient Philosophies

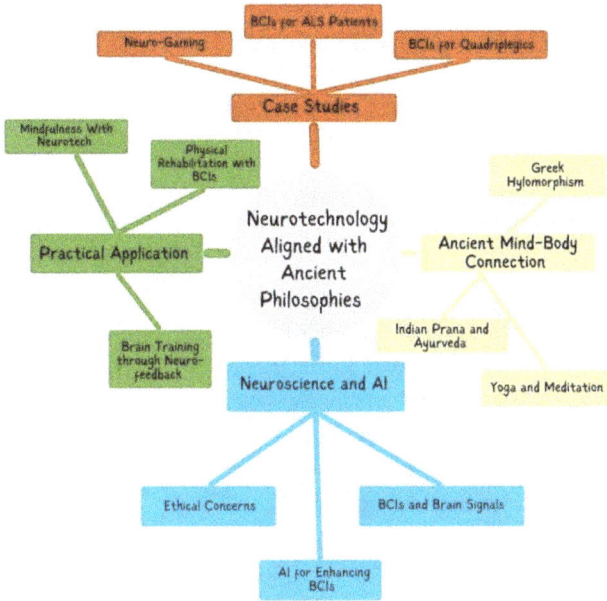

# Chapter 12
# The Ethical Implications of Neuroscience and Ancient Moral Philosophy

## Ethical Dilemmas in Neurotechnology

As neuroscience continues to intersect with cutting-edge technologies like **brain-computer interfaces (BCIs)**, **artificial intelligence (AI)**, and **neurostimulation,** new ethical dilemmas have emerged. These technologies hold immense promise for improving human lives by restoring lost abilities, enhancing cognitive functions, and even exploring new ways of communication. However, with such profound advancements come equally profound concerns about **privacy, autonomy, identity**, and **equity.**

### Privacy and Brain Data

With the development of BCIs and neurostimulation devices, the ability to access and interpret brain data presents a significant ethical challenge. **Neuroprivacy** concerns arise when intimate details of a person's thoughts, intentions, or emotions are potentially exposed through technology. Who owns brain data? Can it be stored, shared, or sold? These questions become increasingly urgent as companies begin to commercialise neurotechnology for consumer use.

### Autonomy and Control

Another critical issue is autonomy. As BCIs allow users to control external devices with their minds, there is a question of whether this technology could lead to external control over the brain. **Neurohacking,** where someone's BCI system could be hacked, raises concerns about autonomy and consent. Furthermore, **cognitive**

**enhancement** technologies may create pressure for individuals to adopt them to remain competitive in their jobs or education, raising questions about **coercion** and **fairness**.

### Identity and Self-Concept

Neurotechnology that enhances memory, focus, or even emotion regulation could blur the lines between human cognition and machine enhancement. This leads to philosophical questions about **what it means to be human**. If we can artificially boost our mental abilities, how does that affect our sense of self? Does altering brain function through external technology diminish the authentic human experience, or does it expand the boundaries of our capabilities?

### Equity and Access

Access to neurotechnology could also exacerbate social inequality. If only the wealthy can afford cognitive enhancements, BCIs, or neurostimulation devices, it could lead to a society where the **cognitively enhanced** have an unfair advantage over those who cannot access these technologies. This could deepen societal divisions and create a **neuro-enhanced elite**. Ethically, ensuring **equitable access** to these technologies is essential to prevent creating cognitive disparities that mirror or amplify existing socioeconomic inequalities.

These dilemmas underscore the need for a robust ethical framework as neuroscience and neurotechnology continue to advance. The intersection of ancient moral philosophies with modern ethical discussions may offer valuable guidance in navigating these complex issues.

## Ancient Moral Philosophies

Ancient civilisations grappled with many of the same moral questions that we face today, albeit without the technological complexities. Yet, the ethical frameworks developed by ancient thinkers offer timeless insights into how we can approach the ethical dilemmas posed by modern neuroscience and neurotechnology.

## Stoicism

Stoic philosophers like **Seneca** and **Epictetus** emphasised the importance of **self-control** and **virtue**. In the context of neurotechnology, Stoicism reminds us of the value of maintaining personal autonomy and avoiding over-reliance on external enhancements for happiness or success. Stoics believed that true contentment comes from within and that external factors, including technologies, should not dictate one's sense of self-worth or virtue. This philosophy encourages us to use neurotechnology mindfully, ensuring that it serves our well-being rather than becoming a crutch.

## Aristotelian Virtue Ethics

**Aristotle** taught that the goal of life is to achieve **eudaimonia**—a state of flourishing through the cultivation of virtues. In terms of neurotechnology, Aristotle's ethics would ask us to consider whether cognitive enhancements or BCIs contribute to or detract from human flourishing. Are we becoming more virtuous, more thoughtful, and more socially responsible through these technologies? The focus here is not just on the outcomes but on the kind of people we are becoming as we integrate technology into our lives.

## Buddhism

Buddhist teachings on **interconnectedness** and **mindfulness** offer essential guidance when considering the ethical implications of neurotechnology. The Buddhist concept of **non-attachment** can be applied to avoid over-identifying with technological enhancements. Buddhism emphasises **self-awareness** and staying grounded in the present moment, suggesting that while technology can be useful, it should not define us or our identity. Additionally, the idea of **compassion** for all beings prompts reflection on how neurotechnology can be used to alleviate suffering rather than deepen societal divides.

**Confucian Ethics**

In **Confucianism**, the focus is on **harmony** and the ethical conduct of individuals within society. Confucian teachings encourage the use of knowledge and technology for the greater good, promoting **social responsibility** and **equity**. In the context of neurotechnology, Confucian thought would urge that these advancements be accessible to all and used in ways that promote collective well-being rather than individual gain. This ethical perspective challenges society to ensure that the benefits of neurotechnology are shared equitably.

These ancient philosophies remind us that, although we live in a technologically advanced world, our ethical challenges are often timeless. The guiding principles of virtue, self-control, mindfulness, and social responsibility are as relevant today in discussions about neurotechnology as they were thousands of years ago.

# Case Studies

### Case Study 1: Cognitive Enhancement and the Ethics of Fairness

David, a 22-year-old college student, begins using a neurostimulation device designed to improve his focus and cognitive processing speed. As he prepares for exams, he finds that the device gives him a significant edge over his classmates, allowing him to absorb information faster and perform better on tests. However, many of his peers cannot afford the technology. David begins to question whether his success is truly based on his hard work or on the enhancement provided by the device.

This case raises ethical concerns about **fairness and access**. If cognitive enhancements are only available to those who can afford them, it could create a competitive imbalance where success is tied to financial resources rather than effort or merit. Ancient philosophies like **Aristotelian ethics** would question whether David's use of the device truly contributes to his personal development or undermines the values of fairness and equity.

**Case Study 2: BCIs and the Loss of Autonomy**

Jane, a patient with **locked-in syndrome**, has regained the ability to communicate through a BCI that interprets her brain signals and converts them into text on a screen. While the technology has significantly improved her quality of life, Jane also feels a sense of dependency on the device. She wonders whether her identity and autonomy are being compromised by her reliance on technology to interact with the world.

This case highlights the ethical dilemma of **autonomy** and **identity**. Although BCIs can restore lost functions, they also create a new form of dependency. Ancient **Stoic philosophy**, which emphasises self-reliance and inner strength, would encourage Jane to reflect on how much control she has over her life and identity in this new relationship with technology. The key ethical question here is whether neurotechnology empowers individuals or subtly diminishes their autonomy.

**Case Study 3: Neuroprivacy and Surveillance**

In a workplace setting, a company introduces neurotechnology to monitor employees' focus and productivity through wearable EEG devices. While the company argues that this will help optimise performance, employees are concerned about their **privacy** and the potential for misuse of their brain data. Could their employer use this data to penalise them for lack of focus or even manipulate their work environment based on their mental states?

This case brings up ethical issues related to **privacy** and **data ownership**. As more neurotechnology enters the commercial sphere, the need for clear regulations about the collection, storage, and use of brain data becomes crucial. **Confucian ethics**, with its focus on harmony and social responsibility, would emphasise the need for transparency, mutual respect, and consent in the use of such technologies, ensuring that they serve the collective good rather than exploiting individuals.

# Practical Reflection

As we face the challenges posed by advancements in neurotechnology, ethical reflection grounded in both modern and ancient wisdom is essential. Here are practical steps and reflections to guide us through these complex issues:

## Balance Technological Use with Inner Growth

It is easy to become overly reliant on external technologies to improve cognitive performance or enhance abilities. However, as **Stoicism** teaches, true growth comes from within. While using neurotechnology, reflect on whether it contributes to your inner development or fosters a dependency that might weaken your autonomy. Regularly engage in practices like meditation or mindfulness to balance technological enhancements with self-awareness and personal growth.

## Ensure Equitable Access

Ancient **Confucian teachings** emphasise the importance of ensuring that technology serves the common good. Advocate for policies that make neurotechnologies accessible to all, preventing the creation of cognitive disparities. Support initiatives that ensure these tools are used to alleviate suffering, restore abilities, and improve the quality of life for those most in need rather than deepening societal divides.

## Protect Neuroprivacy

As neurotechnology becomes more integrated into daily life, it is crucial to demand transparency and regulation around brain data. Just as ancient **Buddhist** philosophy teaches **mindfulness** and **non-attachment**, we must be vigilant in protecting our minds from external surveillance and influence. Support policies that safeguard neuroprivacy, ensuring that individuals maintain control over their cognitive data and how it is used.

## Use Technology to Cultivate Virtue

**Aristotle** taught that the highest purpose of life is to achieve **eudaimonia**, or flourishing, through virtuous living. Reflect on how neurotechnology can help you become a better person—more empathetic, thoughtful, and connected to others. Use these tools not just for personal gain but to contribute to society's well-being, helping others flourish as well.

By integrating these ethical reflections with modern neuroscience and ancient moral wisdom, we can navigate the rapid advancements in neurotechnology with a sense of balance, ensuring that our progress serves both individuals and society in a way that promotes dignity, equity, and human flourishing.

# Summary: The Ethical Implications of Neuroscience and Ancient Moral Philosophy

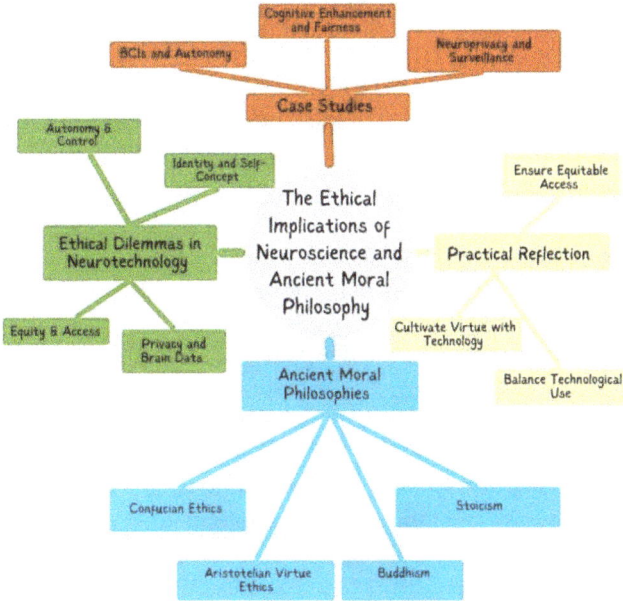

# Glossary

## Chapter 1: The Structure of the Brain and Ancient Theories of Mind

- **Neuron:** A nerve cell that is the fundamental building block of the nervous system, transmitting electrical impulses through synapses.

- **Synapse:** The junction between two neurons where electrical or chemical signals are transmitted.

- **Prefrontal Cortex:** The part of the brain responsible for decision-making, personality expression, and social behaviour.

- **Hippocampus:** A brain region involved in the formation of new memories and spatial navigation.

- **Amygdala:** An almond-shaped structure involved in emotional processing, especially fear and stress.

- **Ancient Theories of Mind:** Historical beliefs about the mind, such as the Egyptian view of the heart as the centre of thought or Indian teachings on balancing mental forces.

## Chapter 2: Neuroplasticity, Cognitive Flexibility, and Ancient Learning Practices

- **Neuroplasticity:** The brain's ability to reorganise and form new neural connections throughout life.

- **Neurogenesis:** The process by which new neurons are created in the brain.

- **Cognitive Flexibility:** The brain's capacity to adapt to new information and shift thinking strategies.

- **Socratic Method:** A form of cooperative argumentative dialogue stimulating critical thinking, used in ancient Greek education.

- **Meditation:** A practice where an individual uses mindfulness to focus on the mind, promoting mental clarity.

# Chapter 3: Depression, Mood, and Ancient Emotional Healing Practices

- **Neurotransmitters:** Chemicals that transmit signals across a synapse from one neuron to another.

- **Serotonin:** A neurotransmitter involved in mood regulation, often linked to feelings of well-being.

- **Dopamine:** A neurotransmitter associated with reward and pleasure systems in the brain.

- **Ayurveda:** An ancient Indian healing system that balances bodily systems using diet, herbal treatments, and yogic breathing.

- **Cognitive Behavioural Therapy (CBT):** A modern psychological treatment that focuses on changing negative thought patterns.

# Chapter 4: Anxiety, Stress, and Ancient Resilience-Building Practices

- **Cortisol:** A hormone released in response to stress, known as the "stress hormone."

- **Fight-or-Flight Response**: The body's automatic response to stress, triggering the release of stress hormones like adrenaline and cortisol.

- **Vagus Nerve**: A major nerve that controls the parasympathetic nervous system, important for stress recovery and relaxation.

- **Qi Gong**: An ancient Chinese practice combining movement, meditation, and controlled breathing to enhance well-being.

- **Mindfulness**: The mental practice of being fully present and aware of one's surroundings, thoughts, and emotions.

# Chapter 5: How We Learn and Ancient Memory Systems

- **Hippocampus**: A region critical for forming and storing memories.

- **Working Memory**: A cognitive system responsible for temporarily holding information available for processing.

- **Mnemonics**: Memory techniques or strategies to aid in the retention of information.

- **Method of Loci**: An ancient mnemonic technique, often called a "Memory Palace," where individuals visualise placing information in specific locations.

- **Oral Tradition**: A form of human communication where knowledge, art, ideas, and cultural material is received and transmitted verbally.

# Chapter 6: Enhancing Cognitive Performance with Focus and Ancient Flow States

- **Flow State**: A mental state of complete immersion and focus in an activity, leading to heightened performance and creativity.

- **Prefrontal Cortex**: Involved in focus and attention regulation, particularly important for sustained concentration.

- **Norepinephrine**: A neurotransmitter that enhances focus, attention, and energy.

- **Yoga**: A physical, mental, and spiritual practice from ancient India that promotes focus and body-mind alignment.

- **Samadhi**: A state of intense concentration and complete absorption, often referred to in ancient yogic texts as the highest form of meditation.

# Chapter 7: Empathy, Compassion, and the Mirror Neuron System in Ancient Contexts

- **Mirror Neurons**: Neurons that fire both when an individual performs an action and when they observe another individual performing the same action, linked to empathy.

- **Theory of Mind**: The ability to attribute mental states—beliefs, intents, desires, emotions—to oneself and others.

- **Emotional Intelligence**: The capacity to recognise, understand, and manage one's own emotions and the emotions of others.

- **Loving-Kindness Meditation**: An ancient Buddhist practice aimed at developing compassion and empathy.

- **Ubuntu**: An ancient African philosophy meaning "I am because we are," emphasising interconnectedness and empathy.

# Chapter 8: Leadership, Influence, and Ancient Philosophical Approaches

- **Oxytocin**: Often referred to as the "love hormone," it plays a role in bonding and trust between individuals.

- **Dopamine**: A neurotransmitter involved in reward, motivation, and leadership behaviour.

- **Stoicism**: An ancient Greek philosophy that teaches resilience and self-control, often employed by leaders to maintain emotional balance.

- **Confucian Leadership**: Rooted in ancient Chinese philosophy, it emphasises moral integrity, social harmony, and leading by example.

- **Mindful Leadership**: A leadership style that integrates mindfulness practices for emotional regulation and decision-making.

# Chapter 9: The Brain-Body Connection and Ancient Holistic Health

- **Autonomic Nervous System**: Controls involuntary functions in the body such as heart rate, digestion, and respiratory rate.

- **Parasympathetic Nervous System**: Part of the autonomic nervous system that promotes relaxation and recovery, often activated by ancient practices like yoga.

- **Qi**: In Chinese philosophy, it is considered the life force that flows through all living things, often associated with health and vitality.

- **Prana**: In Ayurvedic philosophy, the vital life force or energy that sustains physical and mental health.

- **Herbal Medicine**: The use of plant-based substances to treat various health conditions, an ancient practice found across many cultures.

# Chapter 10: Pain Perception and Ancient Pain Management Techniques

- **Chronic Pain**: Long-term pain that persists beyond the normal healing time, often linked to changes in brain pathways.

- **Neurofeedback**: A technique that uses real-time brainwave monitoring to train individuals to self-regulate brain activity, often used for pain management.

- **Acupuncture**: An ancient Chinese medical practice involving the insertion of thin needles into specific points on the body to alleviate pain.

- **Mind-Body Connection**: The interplay between physical sensations and mental processes, particularly in the context of managing pain.

- **Placebo Effect**: The beneficial effect from a treatment that cannot be attributed to the properties of the treatment itself, often linked to belief and expectation.

# Chapter 11: Brain-Computer Interfaces and Neurotechnology Aligned with Ancient Philosophies

- **Brain-Computer Interface (BCI)**: A technology that enables direct communication between the brain and an external device, often used to help individuals with mobility issues.

- **Neural Networks**: Systems of neurons that process information in the brain, which inspire artificial intelligence technologies.

- **Cyborg Ethics**: The ethical implications of merging human biology with technology, especially as related to human enhancement.

- **Mind-Body Unity**: An ancient concept found in many cultures emphasising that the mind and body are not separate entities but one interconnected system.

- **Bionics**: The replacement or enhancement of body parts with mechanical or electronic devices, inspired by biological systems.

# Chapter 12: The Ethical Implications of Neuroscience and Ancient Moral Philosophy

- **Neuroethics**: The field of ethics that studies the implications of neuroscience, especially regarding brain manipulation, enhancement, and privacy.

- **Free Will**: The ability to make choices without coercion, a concept explored both in ancient philosophy and modern neuroscience.

- **Moral Responsibility**: The accountability for one's actions, a concept explored in both neuroscience (how brain functions impact decision-making) and ancient moral philosophies.

- **Utilitarianism**: A moral theory that promotes actions that maximise well-being for the majority, relevant to discussions on neurotechnology's societal impact.

- **Virtue Ethics**: A moral philosophy originating in ancient Greece, focusing on character and moral virtues, relevant to the ethical implications of brain enhancement.

# References

## Chapter 1: The Structure of the Brain and Ancient Theories of Mind

- Albright, T. D., Jessell, T. M., Kandel, E. R., & Posner, M. I. (2000). Neural science: A century of progress and the mysteries that remain. *Neuron, 25*(S1), S1-S55.

- Bear, M. F., Connors, B. W., & Paradiso, M. A. (2015). *Neuroscience: Exploring the 2. Brain* (4th ed.). Wolters Kluwer Health.

- Craig, A. D. (2002). How do you feel? Interoception: The sense of the physiological condition of the body. *Nature Reviews Neuroscience, 3*(8), 655–666.

- Gazzaniga, M. S. (2008). *Cognitive Neuroscience: The Biology of the Mind.* W.W. Norton & Company.

- Kandel, E. R., Schwartz, J. H., & Jessell, T. M. (2013). *Principles of Neural Science* (5th ed.). McGraw-Hill.

## Chapter 2: Neuroplasticity, Cognitive Flexibility, and Ancient Learning Practices

- Doidge, N. (2007). The Brain That Changes Itself: Stories of Personal Triumph from the Frontiers of Brain Science. Penguin.

- Draganski, B., Gaser, C., Busch, V., Schuierer, G., Bogdahn, U., & May, A. (2004). Neuroplasticity: Changes in grey matter induced by training. *Nature, 427*(6972), 311–312.

- Kleim, J. A., & Jones, T. A. (2008). Principles of experience-dependent neural plasticity: Implications for rehabilitation after brain damage. *Journal of Speech, Language, and Hearing Research, 51*(S1), S225-S239.

- Merzenich, M. M. (2013). Soft-Wired: How the New Science of Brain Plasticity Can Change Your Life. Parnassus Publishing.

- Zatorre, R. J., Fields, R. D., & Johansen-Berg, H. (2012). Plasticity in grey and white: Neuroimaging changes in brain structure during learning. *Nature Neuroscience, 15*(4), 528–536.

# Chapter 3: Depression, Mood, and Ancient Emotional Healing Practices

- Allen, N. B., & Badcock, P. B. (2003). The social risk hypothesis of depressed mood: Evolutionary, psychosocial, and neurobiological perspectives. *Psychological Bulletin, 129*(6), 887.

- Drevets, W. C., Price, J. L., & Furey, M. L. (2008). Brain structural and functional abnormalities in mood disorders: Implications for neurocircuitry models of depression. *Brain Structure and Function, 213*(1-2), 93-118.

- Krishnan, V., & Nestler, E. J. (2008). The molecular neurobiology of depression. *Nature, 455*(7215), 894-902.

- Mayberg, H. S. (2009). Targeted electrode-based modulation of neural circuits for depression. *Journal of Clinical Investigation, 119*(4), 717-725.

- Nestler, E. J., Barrot, M., & Dileone, R. J. (2002). Neurobiology of depression. *Neuron, 34*(1), 13-25.

# Chapter 4: Anxiety, Stress, and Ancient Resilience-Building Practices

- Chrousos, G. P., & Gold, P. W. (1992). The concepts of stress and stress system disorders: Overview of physical and behavioural homeostasis. *JAMA, 267*(9), 1244-1252.

- Davidson, R. J., & McEwen, B. S. (2012). Social influences on neuroplasticity: Stress and interventions to promote well-being. *Nature Neuroscience, 15*(5), 689-695.

- McEwen, B. S. (2007). Physiology and neurobiology of stress and adaptation: Central role of the brain. *Physiological Reviews, 87*(3), 873-904.

- Sapolsky, R. M. (2004). Why Zebras Don't Get Ulcers: The Acclaimed Guide to Stress, Stress-Related Diseases, and Coping (3rd ed.). Holt Paperbacks.

- Ulrich-Lai, Y. M., & Herman, J. P. (2009). Neural regulation of endocrine and autonomic stress responses. *Nature Reviews Neuroscience, 10*(6), 397-409.

# Chapter 5: How We Learn and Ancient Memory Systems

- Baddeley, A. (2000). The episodic buffer: A new component of working memory? *Trends in Cognitive Sciences, 4*(11), 417-423.

- Eichenbaum, H. (2004). Hippocampus: Cognitive processes and neural representations that underlie declarative memory. *Neuron, 44*(1), 109-120.

- Scoville, W. B., & Milner, B. (1957). Loss of recent memory after bilateral hippocampal lesions. *Journal of Neurology, Neurosurgery & Psychiatry, 20*(1), 11-21.

- Moser, E. I., Kropff, E., & Moser, M. B. (2008). Place cells, grid cells, and the brain's spatial representation system. *Annual Review of Neuroscience, 31*(1), 69-89.

- Squire, L. R. (2004). Memory systems of the brain: A brief history and current perspective. *Neurobiology of Learning and Memory, 82*(3), 171-177.

# Chapter 6: Enhancing Cognitive Performance with Focus and Ancient Flow States

- Csikszentmihalyi, M. (1990). *Flow: The Psychology of Optimal Experience*. Harper & Row.

- Gazzaley, A., & Rosen, L. D. (2016). The Distracted Mind: Ancient Brains in a High-Tech World. MIT Press.

- Killingsworth, M. A., & Gilbert, D. T. (2010). A wandering mind is an unhappy mind. *Science, 330*(6006), 932.

- Posner, M. I., & Rothbart, M. K. (2007). Research on attention networks as a model for the integration of psychological science. *Annual Review of Psychology, 58*(1), 1-23.

- Raz, A., & Buhle, J. (2006). Typologies of attentional networks. *Nature Reviews Neuroscience, 7*(5), 367-379.

# Chapter 7: Empathy, Compassion, and the Mirror Neuron System in Ancient Contexts

- Decety, J., & Jackson, P. L. (2004). The functional architecture of human empathy. *Behavioural and Cognitive Neuroscience Reviews, 3*(2), 71-100.

- Gallese, V., Keysers, C., & Rizzolatti, G. (2004). A unifying view of the basis of social cognition. *Trends in Cognitive Sciences, 8*(9), 396-403.

- Preston, S. D., & de Waal, F. B. (2002). Empathy: Its ultimate and proximate bases. *Behavioural and Brain Sciences, 25*(1), 1-20.

- Rizzolatti, G., & Craighero, L. (2004). The mirror-neuron system. *Annual Review of Neuroscience, 27*(1), 169-192.

- Singer, T., Seymour, B., O'Doherty, J., Kaube, H., Dolan, R. J., & Frith, C. D. (2004). Empathy for pain involves the affective but not sensory components of pain. *Science, 303*(5661), 1157-1162.

# Chapter 8: Leadership, Influence, and Ancient Philosophical Approaches

- Bass, B. M. (1999). Two decades of research and development in transformational leadership. *European Journal of Work and Organisational Psychology, 8*(1), 9-32.

- Boyatzis, R. E., & McKee, A. (2005). Resonant Leadership: Renewing Yourself and Connecting with Others Through Mindfulness, Hope, and Compassion. Harvard Business Press.

- Goleman, D. (1995). Emotional Intelligence: Why It Can Matter More Than IQ. Bantam Books.

- Rock, D. (2009). Your Brain at Work: Strategies for Overcoming Distraction, Regaining Focus, and Working Smarter All Day Long. HarperCollins.

- Zaccaro, S. J., & Klimoski, R. J. (2001). The Nature of Organisational Leadership: Understanding the Performance Imperatives Confronting Today's Leaders. Jossey-Bass.

# Chapter 9: The Brain-Body Connection and Ancient Holistic Health

- Craig, A. D. (2009). How do you feel—now? The anterior insula and human awareness. *Nature Reviews Neuroscience, 10*(1), 59-70.

- Damasio, A. R. (1994). Descartes' Error: Emotion, Reason, and the Human Brain. G.P. Putnam's Sons.

- McEwen, B. S. (1998). Protective and damaging effects of stress mediators. *New England Journal of Medicine, 338*(3), 171-179.

- Thayer, J. F., & Lane, R. D. (2000). A model of neurovisceral integration in emotion regulation and dysregulation. *Journal of Affective Disorders, 61*(3), 201-216.

- Varela, F. J., Thompson, E., & Rosch, E. (2017). *The Embodied Mind: Cognitive Science and Human Experience.* MIT Press.

# Chapter 10: Pain Perception and Ancient Pain Management Techniques

- Apkarian, A. V., Baliki, M. N., & Geha, P. Y. (2009). Towards a theory of chronic pain. *Progress in Neurobiology, 87*(2), 81-97.

- Eccleston, C., & Crombez, G. (2007). Worry and chronic pain: A misdirected problem-solving model. *Pain, 132*(1-2), 233-236.

- Melzack, R., & Wall, P. D. (1996). Pain mechanisms: A new theory. *Pain Forum, 5*(1), 3-11.

- Moseley, G. L., & Butler, D. S. (2015). Fifteen years of explaining pain: The past, present, and future. *Journal of Pain, 16*(9), 807-813.

- Tracey, I., & Mantyh, P. W. (2007). The cerebral signature for pain perception and its modulation. *Neuron, 55*(3), 377-391.

# Chapter 11: Brain-Computer Interfaces and Neurotechnology Aligned with Ancient Philosophies

- Arguin, M., & Bub, D. N. (1993). Evidence for an independent encoding of spatial relations during transcoding. *Neuropsychologia, 31*(5), 361-376.

- Carmena, J. M., Lebedev, M. A., Crist, R. E., O'Doherty, J. E., Santucci, D. M., Dimitrov, D. F., & Nicolelis, M. A. (2003). Learning to control a brain–machine interface for reaching and grasping by primates. *PLoS Biology, 1*(2), e42.

- Hochberg, L. R., Bacher, D., Jarosiewicz, B., Masse, N. Y., Simeral, J. D., Vogel, J., & Donoghue, J. P. (2012). Reach and grasp by people with tetraplegia using a neurally controlled robotic arm. *Nature, 485*(7398), 372-375.

- Lebedev, M. A., & Nicolelis, M. A. (2006). Brain-machine interfaces: Past, present, and future. *Trends in Neurosciences, 29*(9), 536-546.

- Nicolelis, M. A. (2003). Brain-machine interfaces to restore motor function and probe neural circuits. *Nature Reviews Neuroscience, 4*(5), 417-422.

# Chapter 12: The Ethical Implications of Neuroscience and Ancient Moral Philosophy

- Farah, M. J. (2012). Neuroethics: The ethical, legal, and societal impact of neuroscience. *Annual Review of Psychology, 63*(1), 571-591.

- Greely, H. T., & Wagner, A. D. (2011). Neuroscience-based lie detection: The urgent need for regulation. *American Journal of Bioethics, 11*(2), 38-49.

- Illes, J., & Sahakian, B. J. (Eds.). (2011). *Oxford Handbook of Neuroethics*. Oxford University Press.

- Levy, N. (2008). Introducing neuroethics. *Neuroethics, 1*(1), 1-8.

- Rose, N., & Abi-Rached, J. M. (2013). *Neuro: The New Brain Sciences and the Management of the Mind*. Princeton University Press.

www.ingramcontent.com/pod-product-compliance
Lightning Source LLC
Chambersburg PA
CBHW071238020426
42333CB00015B/1521